Governance of Addictions
European Public Policies

Tamyko Ysa

Joan Colom

Adrià Albareda

Anna Ramon

Marina Carrión

Lidia Segura

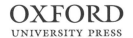
OXFORD
UNIVERSITY PRESS

OXFORD
UNIVERSITY PRESS

Great Clarendon Street, Oxford, OX2 6DP,
United Kingdom

Oxford University Press is a department of the University of Oxford.
It furthers the University's objective of excellence in research, scholarship,
and education by publishing worldwide. Oxford is a registered trade mark of
Oxford University Press in the UK and in certain other countries

Published in the United States of America by Oxford University Press
198 Madison Avenue, New York, NY 10016, United States of America

British Library Cataloguing in Publication Data
Data available

Library of Congress Control Number: 2014935820

ISBN 978–0–19–870330–3

Printed in Great Britain by
Clays Ltd, St Ives plc

Governance
of Addictions

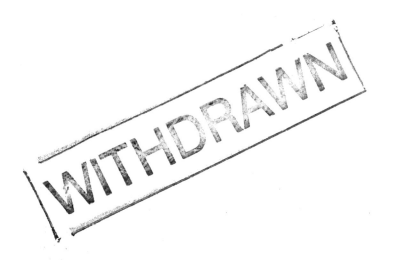

Foreword

This book is the first in a planned series of six arising out of ALICE RAP (Addictions and Lifestyles in Contemporary Europe—Reframing Addictions Project), a five-year, €10-million endeavour co-financed by the Social Sciences and Humanities division of FP7 within the European Commission and led by the Foundation for Biomedical Research based in Barcelona and the Institute of Health and Society in Newcastle University (<http://www.alicerap.eu>). The other planned titles in the Governance of Addictive Substances and Behaviours series are *The Impact of Addictive Substances and Behaviours on Individual and Societal Well-being*; *What Determines Harm from Addictive Substances and Behaviours?*; *Concepts of Addictive Substances and Behaviours across Time and Place*; *The Impact of Market Forces on Addictive Substances and Behaviours*; and *The New Governance of Addictive Substances and Behaviours*.

ALICE RAP studies the place of addictions and lifestyles in contemporary Europe and aims to inform us how we can better redesign their governance. By addictions, we mean the regular and sustained heavy use of drugs such as alcohol, nicotine, and cocaine and regular and sustained heavy engagement in actions such as gambling or internet gaming (Rehm et al. 2013).

There are three potential frames in which we can understand addiction. The first is an evolutionary one. We humans share a co-evolutionary relationship with psychotropic plant substances that is millions of years old (Sullivan and Hagen 2002). These include ethanol in fermenting fruit, ephedrine in khat, arecoline in betel nut, nicotine in various tobacco plants, and cocaine in coca plants. Exposure has both neurotransmitter and nutrient functions and we have the biochemical pathways to metabolize these chemicals. But, of course, exposure was usually only in tiny amounts. The problem is that we are now exposed to these drugs in such huge doses that, for the most part, our bodies and brains do not know how to deal with them in any meaningful way. These drugs also trick our brains into acting as though the benefits of using them far outweigh the harm, whereas this is blatantly not the case. And, of course, a lot of businesses and individuals make a great profit out of this—just think of alcohol and the advertising industry.

The second frame is that when talking about drugs, we should consider not only their relationship with health but also their relationship with societal well-being in its entirety (OECD 2011a). Societal well-being includes many domains that impact on and are impacted by addictive substances—education, work-life balance, productivity, and human capital, to name just a few. But—and for illicit drugs perhaps more importantly—they also impact on personal security, crime, social integration, and transparent governance regimes. As was the case with prohibition of alcohol in the USA during the 1920s, it is the consequence of prohibition, organized crime, and its political influence that has led to many jurisdictions in the Americas, north and south, to call for the abandonment of the prohibition of illicit drugs and adjustment of the existing drug conventions in favour of legal availability managed by government regulations, but still within the frame of global legal agreements.

The third frame is that we grossly underestimate the harm done by addictive drugs. Let's take alcohol as an example, the only psychoactive drug not subject to a legally binding agreement. Alcohol was the world's fifth most important risk factor for ill-health and premature death in 2010, after high blood pressure, tobacco, household air pollution from cooking fires, and a diet low in fruit, moving up from eighth position in 1990 (Lim et al. 2012). The annual social costs of alcohol from impaired health, crime, and lost productivity work out at about €300 for every single EU citizen, man, woman, and child (Rehm et al. 2012). It is estimated that this would likely double to about €600 for every one of us, if the social costs that alcohol causes to people surrounding the drinker are included—friends, families, colleagues, and strangers (Laslett et al. 2010). Much of these costs are preventable and ill-affordable in times of economic downturn.

There are three groups of action that can inform better governance of addictions. The first is to capitalize on the importance of social networks. Data from the US Framingham Heart Study found that at any one time, for every additional contact among family and friends who chose not to drink alcohol, the next time an individual was asked, the likelihood of heavy drinking was reduced by ten per cent (Rosenquist et al. 2010). Likewise, for every additional contact among friends and family who drank heavily—more than one drink (women) or two drinks (men) a day—the next time an individual was asked, they were 18 per cent more likely to drink heavily.

The second action is to recognize that changing the social and physical environment is far more effective in helping people improve their health than trying to change individual behaviour alone. Social and physical changes that take the healthiest route are the easiest to follow. This means that government action is absolutely essential. There are powers only governments can exercise, policies only governments can mandate and enforce, and results only governments can achieve. Governments at all levels can regulate the markets in which private businesses operate through mechanisms that impact particularly on price, availability, and advertising (World Economic Forum and WHO 2011). One of the biggest impediments of governments putting health as their paramount concern is a default in the democratic process and their unwillingness or inability to stand up to big tobacco and big alcohol.

The third action is to develop better metrics. ALICE RAP is developing a tool for managing the harm done by addictions, with the development of a footprint of nations, regions and cities, sectors and organizations, and products and services to promote accountability and monitor change. Modelled on a carbon footprint (Williams et al. 2012), an addictions footprint would measure, for example, the amount of alcohol-related ill-health and premature death resulting from the actions of an entity or organization, such as introducing a minimum price per gram of alcohol by a government, bringing forward pub closing times in a city, or from the amount of beer produced in different markets by the world's largest brewer.

If you want to redesign the governance of addictions, it is vital to identify the starting point, and this book does just that. This is the first time that this has ever been done in such a thorough and comprehensive way. And the findings are remarkable. In addictions policies, the structure of the approach follows the strategy of the approach. Countries that implement a well-being and relational management strategy tend to embrace a comprehensive policy for addictions. They also tend to be those in which the Ministry of Health, as opposed to the Ministry of the Interior, is the main body responsible for planning and implementing drug policy. They have a harm-reduction as opposed to a regulatory approach; decriminalize rather than criminalize drug use; have proactive rather than post-factum policy-making; have a health-oriented rather than a public-security approach; and aim to protect the public and society in general rather than focus on individual responsibility. Countries that embrace a comprehensive policy for addictions tend to tackle legal and illicit substances together, as opposed to split substance policies; have a long experience in drug and addiction policies, as opposed to little experience and poor continuity; have complex rather than simple organizational structures; have multi-level governance and high levels of devolution, rather than centralized organizational structures; and involve rather than exclude stakeholders.

Since only just over one-quarter of the twenty-eight European countries studied fall in the well-being and relational management strategy/comprehensive policy for addictions cluster, there is clearly an enormous opportunity for improvement for Europe as a whole. And there are no excuses for not seizing this opportunity—this book lays out the clear elements of what would constitute better policy.

Peter Anderson
International Coordinator of the ALICE RAP project; Chief Series Editor, Governance of Addictive Substances and Behaviours; Professor, Substance Use, Policy and Practice, Newcastle University, England; Professor, Alcohol and Health, Maastricht University, Netherlands

Acknowledgements

The authors want to thank the 7th European Framework for funding this research and all the people involved in the ALICE RAP project for their support, comments, and contributions over the past few years. We would especially like to thank Peter Anderson, Toni Gual, and all the team from the Hospital Clínic of Barcelona for being excellent facilitators and providing the support we needed to reach our desired goals.

We would like to express our special thanks to Lourdes Feans for the collection, management, and analysis of the mass media information, and to Xavier Fernández-i-Marín for his sound methodological approach to analysing our quantitative results. We are also in debt to Jan-Erik Karlsen for his contributions to the research meetings as well as his revisions of draft chapters, which were remarkably valuable. We cannot forget Xavier Majó, who made a special contribution to this work by participating in specific meetings, solving doubts, and providing much-appreciated ideas and new ways of approaching this research. Neither must we forget the help of Oriol Iglesias, marketing professor, in conducting the naming session that led to the different labels used in the book. As a collaborative project, this book could not have been done without the help and contributions of our area partners in ALICE RAP; special thanks to Franz Trautmann, Esa Österberg, Thomas Karlsson, and Mikaela Lindeman, whose work has been especially useful to this study.

We would also like to thank all the people who have participated in interviews and/or revised our work: Joseph Barry, Gerhard Bühringer, Pieter de Coninck, Fernanda Feijao, Vibeke Asmussen Frank, Sir Ian Gilmore, Cees Goos, Matilda Hellman, John Holmes, Eric Janssen, Matej Kosir, David P. Martínez Oró, Maurice Mittelmark, David Nutt, Esa Österberg, Dag Rekve, Robin Room, Emanuele Scafato, Sir Jack Stewart-Clark, Franz Trautman, and Witold Zatonski.

Last but, as usual, not least, we would like to thank to all our colleagues from ESADE and GENCAT for their patience and support throughout this project.

Contents

List of contributors *xv*

Abbreviations *xvi*

1 Introduction to European public policies *1*

    1.1   Presentation *1*

    1.2   Addiction: A growing global concern *1*

    1.3   The long road that led us here *3*

    1.4   Governance of addictions: A wicked issue *6*

    1.5   The structure of this book *7*

2 Methodology to analyse governance on addictions in Europe *9*

    2.1   Introduction to governance of addictions *9*

    2.2   Departing from existing country comparative analysis in Europe: Contextual indicators *9*

    2.3   Information gathering for governance of addictions *11*

    2.4   Triangulation of sources of information *17*

    2.5   Governance of addictions in Europe *19*

    2.6   European models of governance of addictions *19*

    2.7   Cluster analysis of addiction policies in Europe *22*

    2.8   Challenges and limitations of the research *24*

3 European Union achievements and the role of international organizations *27*

    3.1   Introduction to EU policy on addictions *27*

    3.2   The EU addiction policy process: A historical perspective *27*

    3.3   Stakeholder involvement in EU policy-making on addictions *36*

    3.4   Impact of addictive substances and geopolitics in European regions and countries *38*

    3.5   The leading and coordinating role of international organizations *41*

    3.6   EU achievements: Main common features of the member states' policies *42*

    3.7   Conclusion: The EU process. Seeking convergence *44*

4 Model 1: Trendsetters in illicit substances (Belgium, Czech Republic, Germany, Italy, Luxembourg, the Netherlands, Portugal, Spain) *47*

    4.1   Introduction to Model 1 *47*

4.2 Description of the model: Approaches to the governance of addictions *47*

4.3 Germany *50*

4.4 Belgium *52*

4.5 The Czech Republic *54*

4.6 Italy *56*

4.7 Luxembourg *58*

4.8 The Netherlands *59*

4.9 Portugal *61*

4.10 Spain *65*

4.11 Conclusion to Model 1 in Europe *67*

5 Model 2: Regulation of legal substances (Finland, France, Ireland, Norway, Sweden, UK) 69

5.1 Description of the model: Approaches to the governance of addictions *69*

5.2 Sweden *74*

5.3 Finland *77*

5.4 France *79*

5.5 Ireland *81*

5.6 The UK *83*

5.7 Norway *85*

5.8 Conclusion to Model 2 in Europe *86*

6 Model 3: Transitioning (Austria, Bulgaria, Cyprus, Denmark, Poland, Slovenia) 89

6.1 Description of the model: Approaches to the governance of addictions *89*

6.2 Poland *90*

6.3 Austria *92*

6.4 Bulgaria *94*

6.5 Cyprus *96*

6.6 Denmark *97*

6.7 Slovenia *98*

6.8 Conclusion to Model 3 in Europe *100*

7 Model 4: The traditional approach (Estonia, Greece, Hungary, Latvia, Lithuania, Malta, Romania, Slovakia) 103

7.1 Description of the model: Approaches to the governance of addictions *103*

7.2 Slovakia *105*

7.3 Estonia *107*

7.4   Greece *109*

7.5   Hungary *110*

7.6   Latvia *111*

7.7   Lithuania *113*

7.8   Malta *114*

7.9   Romania *115*

7.10 Conclusion to Model 4 in Europe *116*

8 Conclusion: The key to understanding the governance of addictions
in Europe *119*

8.1   European government policies on addictions: A comparative
analysis *119*

8.2   Governance framework and trends *120*

8.3   Four models of governance of addictions in Europe *123*

8.4   The contingent comparative approach to addictions *126*

8.5   Research limitations *127*

8.6   Final remarks *127*

Annexes *131*

Bibliography *218*

Index *238*

List of contributors

Adrià Albareda MSc in International Relations and BA in Political Science. Researcher in the Institute for Public Governance and Management at ESADE Business School. He is working on research projects on governance, public management, management of networks, and public–private partnerships.

Marina Carrión BA in Political Science. She is currently working as a researcher at the Public Health Department of the Government of Catalonia.

Joan Colom Doctor of Medicine, Executive Master in Public Management (ESADE Business School), and Master in Addiction (University of Barcelona). He is the Director of the Programme on Substance Abuse at the Catalan Agency of Public Health of the Government of Catalonia, and Advisor to the World Health Organization. He is the recipient of the Queen Sofía Award for prevention of substances abuse.

Anna Ramon PhD in Sociology at the University of Barcelona. Her thesis is entitled 'The Structure and Dynamics of Social Capital in Europe'. She is currently working as a researcher at the Public Health Department of the Government of Catalonia and is an Associate Professor at the University of Barcelona.

Lidia Segura Clinical psychologist, addiction, and public health specialist. She is the coordinator of the implementation of policies and prevention programmes on alcohol in Catalonia.

Tamyko Ysa PhD in Political Science, Executive Master in Public Management, MSc in Public Administration and Public Policies (LSE), BA in Political Science, and BA in Law. Associate Professor in the Department of Strategy and General Management and in the Institute for Public Governance and Management at ESADE Business School (<http://www.esade.edu/public>), serving also as a visiting researcher in the Department of Business and Politics at Copenhagen Business School.

Abbreviations

ACMD	Advisory Council on the Misuse of Drugs of the United Kingdom
AIDS	Acquired immunodeficiency syndrome
ALICE RAP	Addiction and Lifestyles in Contemporary Europe—Reframing Addictions Project
AMPHORA	Alcohol Measures for Public Health Research Alliance
ANDT	Alcohol, Narcotic drugs, Doping, and Tobacco
APA	American Psychological Association
APTA	Alcohol Produces and Traders Association of Latvia
ASAM	American Society of Addiction Medicine
AU	Austria
BAC	Blood alcohol content
BE	Belgium
BoE	Brewers of Europe
BU	Bulgaria
BUMAD	Belarus, Ukraine, Moldova Action Drug Programme
CAC	Cyprus Anti-Drugs Council
CADAP	Central Asia Drug Action Programme
CARICC	Central Asian Regional Information and Coordination Centre
CCDA	Hungarian Coordination Committee on Drug Affairs
CECCM	Confederation of European Community Cigarette Manufacturers
CEE	Council of the European Communities
CEEC	Central and Eastern European Countries
CEEV	Comité Européen des Entreprises Vins
CELAD	European Committee to Combat Drugs
CIA	Central Intelligence Agency
CND	Commission on Narcotic Drugs
COREPER	Committee of Permanent Representatives
CPI	Corruption Perception Index
CSF	European Civil Society Forum on Drugs
CY	Cyprus
CZ	Czech Republic
DAG	Drug Advisory Group of Ireland
DE	Germany
DG	Directorate-General
DG JUSTICE	Directorate-General for Justice
DG SANCO	Directorate-General for Health and Consumers
DHMA	Danish Health and Medicines Authority
DK	Denmark
EAHC	Executive Agency for Health and Consumers
EC	European Commission
ECB	European Central Bank
ECMA	European Cigar Manufacturers Association
ECTR	European Confederation of Tobacco Retailers
ECU	European Currency Unit
EDU	Europol Drugs Unit
EEC	European Economic Community

EFRD	European Forum for Responsible Drinking
EMA	European Medicines Agency
EMCDDA	European Monitoring Centre for Drugs and Drug Addictions
ENCOD	European Coalition for Just and Effective Drug Policies
EP	European Parliament
EPHA	European Public Health Alliance
ES	Estonia
ESTA	European Smoking Tobacco Association
EU	European Union
EURAD	Europe against Drugs
EUROCARE	European Alcohol Policy Alliance
EUROJUST	European Union's Judicial Cooperation Unit
EUROPOL	European Union's law enforcement agency
FCTC	Framework Convention of Tobacco Control
FDCO	Federal Drug Coordination Office
FDF	Federal Drug Forum
FI	Finland
FP7	Seventh Framework Programme
FR	France
GDP	Gross domestic product
GR	Greece
HDG	Horizontal Drugs Group
HIV	Human immunodeficiency virus infection
HU	Hungary
ICD	International Classification of Diseases
ICDL	Inter-ministerial Commission on Drugs of Luxembourg
IDPC	International Drug Policy Consortium

IDT	Institute on Drugs and Drug Addiction of Portugal (*Instituto da Droga e da Toxicodependência*)
IDU	Injecting drug users
IMF	International Monetary Fund
INCB	International Narcotics Control Board
IR	Ireland
IT	Italy
JHA	Justice and Home Affairs
LT	Lithuania
LU	Luxembourg
LV	Latvia
MDMA	Methylenedioxy-*N*-Methylamphetamine
MEP	Members of the European Parliament
MILDT	Inter-departmental Mission for the Fight against Drugs and Drug Addiction (*Mission interministérielle de lutte contre la drogue et la toxicomanie*)
MT	Malta
NAA	Anti-drug Agency of Romania
NGO	Non-governmental organization
NHS	National Health Service
NIS	newly independent states
NL	Netherlands
NO	Norway
NordAN	Nordic Alcohol and Drug Policy Network
NSP	needle and syringe programme
NSPDA	National Strategy for Prevention of Drug Addiction of Estonia
ÖBIG	REITOX Focal Point Austria
OECD	Organization for Economic Co-operation and Development

OFDT	French Monitoring Centre for Drugs and Drug Addiction (*Observatoire français des drogues et des toxicomanies*)
OKANA	Organization against drugs of Greece
OLAF	European Anti-Fraud Office
OST	Opioid substitution treatment
PL	Poland
PT	Portugal
REITOX	European Information Network on Drugs and Drug Addiction (*Réseau Européen d'information sur les drogues et les toxicomanies*)
RO	Romania
SCAD	South Caucasus Action Drug Programme
SELEC	South-East Law Enforcement Centre
SGI	sustainable governance indicators
SK	Slovakia
SL	Slovenia
SMG	Narcotic Substances Act of Austria (*Suchtmittelgesetz*)
SNBHW	Swedish National Board of Health and Welfare (*Socialstyrelsen*)
SNIPH	Swedish National Institute of Public Health (*Statensfolkhälsoinstitut*)
SP	Spain
STAKES	National Research and Development Centre for Welfare and Health (*Sosiaali-ja Terveysalan Tutkimus-ja Kehittämiskeskus*)
SW	Sweden
TI	Transparency International
UK	United Kingdom
UMHRI	University Mental Health Research Institute
UN	United Nations
UNAIDS	Joint United Nations Programme on HIV/AIDS
UNGASS	United Nations General Assembly
UNODC	United Nations Office on Drugs and Crime
USA	United States of America
USSR	Union of Soviet Socialist Republics
WB	World Bank
WHO	World Health Organization
WVS	World Values Survey

Chapter 1

Introduction to European public policies

1.1 Presentation

More than one hundred years ago, on 23 January 1912, the first international convention on drugs, intended comprehensively to tackle drug control, was signed in The Hague. A century later, despite the efforts made on all levels by numerous actors and all the knowledge and evidence amassed, our society is still struggling to find ways to deal effectively with addictive substances and behaviours and, even harder, to reach global consensus on the issue. Why is governance of addiction so difficult? What can we learn from recent experiences and efforts in Europe? Is it possible to talk about the existence of different typologies of governance of addiction in Europe? Is there a European model of governance of addiction? This book aims to respond to these questions and presents the state of the art in the governance of addictions in the twenty-seven European Union member states, plus Norway. Current approaches to governing addictive substances are reviewed to show what can be learned from them in order to reframe the governance of addiction.

This book presents comparative multidisciplinary research (including public management, health, political science, sociology, economics, and law) that develops an explanatory framework for understanding how governments formulate and implement addiction policies in Europe. For this purpose, four substances are taken into account: heroin, cannabis, alcohol, and tobacco. The study focuses on policies and governance practices in Europe from the beginning of 2005 to the end of 2011. However, to provide a historical perspective and overview of the evolution of governance, documents from 1980 to 2012 have been taken into account.

1.2 Addiction: A growing global concern

In a consumerist and globalized Europe, during a hitherto unknown period of peace, new lifestyles have emerged over the last fifty years, as have new and not always pleasant forms of relationship and coexistence with addictive substances. In Europe each year there are around 8,500 drug-related deaths, 2,100 of which

---

This book was finished before Croatia became a EU member state.

are from HIV/AIDS attributable to drug use, while 3,000 people become infected with HIV because of drug use (EC-DG Justice 2012). Furthermore, 120,000 people aged between 15 and 64 die every year in Europe because of alcohol consumption, and alcohol costs about €300 a year per person in terms of productivity loss, health, and criminality (ALICE–RAP 2012). Tobacco consumption causes the death of 695,000 people between 35 and 69 years old every year, the largest single cause of avoidable death in the EU (EC-DG Health 2012). In summary, around 800,000 people die every year due to substance consumption, which represents 0.16 per cent of the total population of the twenty-eight countries from which we drew our data. It is worth noting that young people and disadvantaged groups are among those more affected, which adds even more complexity to the issue and makes it, if possible, even more essential to look for feasible responses and solutions. Apart from fatal consequences, addictions also cause further harm to users, their relatives and friends, and to society as a whole. This has generated a growing concern and a joint mobilization of civil society and governments to find ways to tackle this issue seriously.

Notwithstanding that, what should we understand by 'addiction'? Is this the best term to use when addressing governance issues? How does the addiction debate affect governance? There have been many attempts throughout history to define the term 'addiction', and it is not our intention to enter into that debate here. However, it is necessary to provide some background about what can be understood by addiction and what are the current trends. As Berridge and Mars (2004: 747) note, 'addiction is a contested term, first in widespread use in medicine in the early twentieth century to describe compulsive drug taking. Replaced older language of "habit", "inebriety", or "morphinomania". Initially focused on alcohol and drugs, but latterly applied to nicotine, symbolising "ownership" by public health as well as by psychiatry.' In this regard, in the 1950s the World Health Organization (WHO) distinguished drug habituation from drug addiction on the basis of the absence of physical dependence, desire rather than compulsion to take the drug, and little or no tendency to increase the dose. Later, in the 1960s, WHO recommended that both terms should be abandoned in favour of 'dependence', which can exist in various degrees of severity. The latest (tenth) International Classification of Diseases (WHO 2010) promoted by WHO still excludes the term 'addiction'.

However, the concept of addiction continues to be widely employed by professionals and the general public alike. In contrast to WHO's position, the American Psychological Association (APA) still uses the term 'addictions' as a feasible umbrella to cover both psychological and physical symptoms of dependence and thus addictive behaviours. And the American Society of Addiction Medicine (ASAM) states that addiction is a chronic neurological disorder involving many brain functions, most notably a devastating imbalance in the so-called reward circuitry.

As noted by Rehm et al. (2013), these terms are to a certain extent outdated, and there is a need to find a new term that properly reflects the magnitude of the issue, its causes, and consequences. More specifically, the authors propose the term 'heavy use over time', which is responsible, among other things, for changes in the brain and other physiological characteristics of substance use disorders, intoxication, and withdrawal and tolerance phenomena—regarded as central to current definitions of addiction or dependence. Furthermore, 'heavy use over time' is the main origin of social consequences arising from substance use disorders, such as problems fulfilling social roles. Finally, it is responsible for the greater part of the substance-attributable burden of disease and mortality. In short, this definition embraces the object of analysis of this book and eliminates some of the current problems and operationalizations.

In this book, we look at public policies dealing with the addicted population but we also take into account strategies aimed at controlling or regulating consumption of addictive substances in general, use and abuse of drugs (including recreational drug use), intoxication, and detoxification and rehabilitation. We address a range of issues from manufacturing, trafficking, possession, and consumption to prevention, treatment, and social reintegration of affected individuals and their immediate environment.

1.3 The long road that led us here

Although human beings have always consumed drugs, the patterns and the substances we use nowadays are not the same as they were a hundred years ago. The 'traditional' ways of consuming addictive substances have historically been linked to social, liturgical, and cultural factors. However, after the industrial revolution and the consequent evolution of social organization, the relationship with drugs changed: addictive substance consumption expanded considerably and become more linked to leisure time (Pavarini 1983). Moreover, following Díaz (1998), there are different historical factors that contributed to the current consumerist model of drugs, among which the development of the pharmaceutical industry, the emergence of chemical addictive compounds, and the process of globalization are determinant.

Three general trends on how addictions have been tackled by Western European governments can be identified: the moral paradigm, assistentialism, and the public-health approach. The moral paradigm emerged at the beginning of the twentieth century as a reactive and puritan response to the popularization of drugs, and promoted a moral crusade against them. This approach considered drug consumption as an indication of individual weakness and lack of self-control. The moral attitude was both to stigmatize and 'save' drug consumers, who were viewed as sinful and vicious. Treatment was mainly provided either by 'beneficiary houses' or by health professionals, who a few decades later embraced an assistentialist approach. The moral paradigm was especially promoted in the USA by the temperance movements. The temperance movements were social movements urging the prohibition of alcohol beverages. An example was the American Temperance Society, founded in 1826, which had as one of its slogans 'Lips that touch liquor shall not touch ours.' The main achievement of the temperance movements in the USA was the 1920 constitutional amendment limiting the sale, manufacture, and transportation of alcohol for consumption—the 'Dry Law'. The temperance movements exported this approach through conferences, conventions, and international agreements (Shanghai 1909; The Hague 1912, 1913, and 1914; and Geneva 1925, 1931, and 1936). The last of these conventions, Geneva 1936, implied that signatory members accepted the prohibitionist approach promoted by the USA.

The moral paradigm partially persisted through UN conventions into the second half of the twentieth century—the Single Convention (1961) as amended by the 1972 protocol, the Convention on Psychotropic Substances (1971), and the Convention Against Illicit Traffic in Narcotic Drugs and Psychotropic Substances (1988) (Courtwright 2001). However, its current relevance is only residual, especially in Europe where the temperance movement has never been as strong as in the USA.

The new economic model that emerged after the Second World War, the development of the welfare state in Western Europe, and a growing middle class are key factors to understanding the emergence of the assistentialist paradigm. As noted by Romaní (1997), during the 1950s and 1960s the drugs phenomenon was consolidated as a characteristic of complex societies and the drugs consumerist model was reified. In this context, the scientific view that prevailed considered drug consumers to be diseased, and dependence to be an illness that had to be treated from a medical scientific approach. Treatments were based on prescription and abstinence, and relapse was considered a failure. This approach established a power relation between the physician and the patient (Foucault 1963), the former representing knowledge and the latter considered an outsider whom science had to heal. It was also in this period that the WHO started promoting international treaties (the first in 1961) considering drug consumers as outcasts from modern societies.

The public-health approach emerged hand in hand with the heroin and cocaine boom during the 1970s and 1980s. The popularization of heroin consumption in particular represented a turning point in public-health and security problems. At first, most countries opted for an assistance strategy, with the ultimate aim of total abstinence by the patient. However, the emergence of HIV/AIDS forced a change of attitude and governments introduced health-oriented measures, the most important of which were harm reduction programmes. For instance, in 1982 drug users forced Amsterdam city council to set up the first needle and syringe exchange programme, to prevent a hepatitis B epidemic among injecting drug users (Burning 1991). And in 1988, the scientific advisory body of the UK government stated that the 'spread of HIV is a greater danger to individual and public health than drug misuse' (Advisory Council on the Misuse of Drugs 1988).

Although the public-health approach had the same goals as the assistentialist one—total abstinence—it also embedded intermediate goals focusing on preserving health and improving the quality of life of drug consumers. As Rhodes and Hedrich (2010: 19) show, 'a core principle of harm reduction is the development of pragmatic responses to dealing with drug use through a hierarchy of intervention goals that place primary emphasis on reducing the health-related harms of continued drug use'. Despite the efforts of this model to avoid the stigmatization of heroin consumers, negative public opinion towards this group of people did not change during the 1980s and the 1990s and still persists today. To fight stigmatization and discrimination, users themselves started to organize in different countries. The Junkie Unions in the late 1970s in the Netherlands were probably the first organizations to fight for users' rights (Van Dam 2007).

During the 1990s the heroin alarm became less prevalent in Western Europe not only because consumption was significantly reduced, but also because of the emergence of cocaine and new synthetic and designer drugs. In contrast, during the same decade Eastern European countries (former satellites of the USSR) experienced the scourge of heroin that Western European countries had been through in the 1980s. Furthermore, the 1990s were characterized as the decade in which problematic use of alcohol, associated with high-risk consumption patterns among young people, emerged.

In this context, recreational consumption of legal and illicit substances avoided stigmatization, which only appeared when consumption was problematic. Consumption became normalized and was no longer linked to marginal contexts (Romaní 2009). Therefore, for broad social sectors drug consumption became socially accepted and part of the hegemonic cultural model. The twenty-first century began with the diffusion of drug and polydrug consumption, especially of alcohol, cannabis, cocaine, methylenedioxy-N-methylamphetamine (MDMA), and crystal meth. Nowadays, consumption of drugs is an activity in itself for young people; it does not require any kind of justification and is compatible with any recreational activity (Díaz et al. 2004).

Bearing in mind the diversity of consumption scenarios, its progressive normalization in some contexts, and even its trivialization in others, Western societies have been forced to find renewed policies and adapt better to these realities, some of which are nothing more than old policies with a modern look. Nowadays, European public policies on addiction are characterized by three trends (Trautmann 2013) that can co-exist at both national and European levels.

The first trend, decriminalization of drug use, is especially relevant for illicit drugs like cannabis and heroin. This is characterized as a health-oriented approach that no longer regards drug consumers as criminals but as patients. In parallel, consumption and/or possession of small amounts for personal use are treated as misdemeanours and not as criminal offences. The second trend is the wider introduction of harm reduction policies for both illicit and legal substances. Harm reduction appeared as a practice with the heroin boom of the 1980s and the consequent need to find ways to deal with its consequences. Since the beginning of the 2000s, acceptance of harm reduction has significantly increased among European countries, has been embraced by international organizations such as the EU, the WHO, and the UN, and is recognized as a characteristic of public-health-oriented policies. The third trend is a shift from repression towards regulation. This trend has been the main approach to dealing with legal substances like alcohol and tobacco, but has also recently been developed for cannabis in different countries.

1.4 **Governance of addictions: A wicked issue**

In the last three decades, the complexity of dealing with public policies has increased, mainly due to what are known as 'wicked problems' (Rittel and Webber 1973), which by definition are inherently resistant to clear and agreed solutions. As Kickert et al. (1997), Stoker (1998), Bovaird (2004), Mendoza and Vernis (2008), Esteve et al. (2012b), and Ysa et al. (2014) state, 'the need to respond to 'wicked social problems' requires public agencies to be prepared to work in partnership with other public, civil society, and business organizations' (Mendoza and Vernis 2008: 392). Moreover, Lozano et al. (2006: 392) add that 'the governance of our complex and interdependent societies will not be possible unless we turn the sense of responsibility among their many social actors into one of co-responsibility'. Hence public, private, and non-profit sectors come together to address issues, solve problems, and provide services that are too complex and/or costly for any organization to handle on its own (O'Toole 1997).

Governance is understood as 'the processes and structures of public policy decision-making and management that engage people constructively across the boundaries of public agencies, levels of government, and/or the public, private and civic spheres in order to carry out a public purpose that could not otherwise be accomplished' (Emerson et al. 2012: 2). Complex societies have boosted governance as a necessary process to tackle wicked problems. Nonetheless, governments still have a major role to play within the governance process as they retain critical tasks that cannot be delegated to other sectors, such as steering and defining strategies. In this sense, policy is still one of the main tools for influencing and shaping the governance of addictions and for this reason is one of the main foci of this book.

The complexity of addiction issues leaves no doubt that they represent a wicked issue that must be tackled by different levels of government in collaboration with NGOs and businesses. The governance of addiction is a recognized complex area that does not follow the traditional linear model (problem—options—solution—implementation) and is influenced by various factors that intervene in policy-making, due to its implications for society and the controversy that it generates (Ritter and Bammer 2010). As a result, we deal with policies that are 'co-produced by a wide range of actors at the level of the state (ministries, parliaments, agencies, authorities, and commissions), society (businesses, citizens, community groups, global media including networked social media, foundations) and supranationally (the European Union, the United Nations)' (WHO 2011b: viii). The governance of addiction is also influenced by many stakeholders from different fields: health, justice, public order, safety, economy, trade, etc. This wide range of stakeholders, and the international domain related to drug trafficking and the EU, make the governance of addictions even more complex.

A further matter of complexity to add to the addictions issue is the role of traditions, national cultures, and ideological rhetoric. In Europe this means that we do not find the same unified response to alcohol, and rejection of it, as we do for other substances. There is a double standard relating to illicit and legal substances and stigma is traditionally associated with drug consumers. Regarding ideological rhetoric, the addictions policy is heavily impacted by the turnover of political parties, which is easy to see through the time discontinuities in strategy and makes it difficult to set sustained responses in motion.

1.5 **The structure of this book**

In Chapter 2 we present the methodological design for the study research. Subsequently, we analyse international trends, with a special focus on the role of the

EU and its governance of addictions model. The aim of Chapter 3 is to analyse how the EU and its policies influence the twenty-seven member states, plus Norway. In Chapters 4 to 7 we present the four approaches to governing addictions in Europe. The final chapter contains our conclusions and thoughts on future prospects.

Chapter 2

Methodology to analyse governance on addictions in Europe

2.1 Introduction to governance of addictions

In this chapter we present the methodology used for this research in order to develop a comprehensive analysis and put forward the state of the art of the governance of addictions in the twenty-seven EU member states, plus Norway. The study is a combination of qualitative and quantitative analysis. For two years, we have gathered information from these countries to analyse their governance of addictions. The research process is built from a bottom-up approach, by collecting data on each country and then looking at the commonalities among the countries to classify them.

In a nutshell, our book started by gathering information on all twenty-eight countries. For each of the countries a table and a report were built, logging key information about the country. This information was complemented with semi-structured interviews and a survey with experts in the field.

2.2 Departing from existing country comparative analysis in Europe: Contextual indicators

Since our intention is to research whether there is a single European model for addictions or several, we depart from comparative studies that classify countries using variables that are keys for public policies on addictions. Those are: Esping-Andersen's welfare states regimes, the OECD Better Life Initiative, sustainable governance indicators, world values survey data, and Corruption Perception Index indicators (Esping-Andersen 1990; Ferrera 1996; Hall and Soskice 2001; Bohle and Greskovits 2006). Esping-Andersen (1990: 80), defines the welfare state as:

> the institutional arrangements, rules and understandings that guide and shape current social policy decisions, expenditure developments, problem definitions, and even the respond-and-demand structure of citizens and welfare consumers. The existence of policy regimes reflects the circumstance that short term policies, reforms, debate, and

decision-making take place within frameworks of historical institutionalization that differ qualitatively between countries.

The policy interest in well-being has grown in the last ten years and, in 2008, the French government convened the Stiglitz Commission—Commission on the Measurement of Economic Performance and Social Progress—(Stiglitz et al. 2009), aimed at measuring economic performance and social progress. The final report in 2009 highlighted the impermanence of subjective measures of quality of life when trying to gauge the overall well-being and progress of a society, and encouraged governments to collect these subjective measures of quality of life. Since then, well-being and progress have been incorporated in different governmental agendas, and the OECD has made remarkable achievements in this field by creating the Better Life Initiative to measure quality of life (OECD 2011c). The added value of this framework is the inclusion of subjective measures to obtain a view of the quality-of-life status in a country. This is needed since traditional indicators, such as GDP, do not reflect the actual differences in society further than gross product per capita.

The OECD Better Life Initiative measurement system takes into account material living conditions and quality of life. Each block includes variables to measure well-being and progress. Specifically, the variables we used for this book include material living conditions (housing, income, and jobs) and quality of life (community, education, environment, governance, health, life satisfaction, safety, and work-life balance). These variables provide us with the state of the art of OECD countries, presenting their weaknesses and their strengths. From a methodological point of view, the main limitation in using the OECD indicators is that some EU countries—Latvia, Lithuania, Romania, Bulgaria, Cyprus, and Malta—are not OECD members.

We complemented the OECD Better Life Initiative with two sustainable governance indicators. The first is the status index, which examines each state's reform needs in terms of the quality of democracy and performance in key policy fields (Bertelsmann Stiftung 2011). More specifically, it analyses the quality of democracy and policy performance in areas such as economy and employment, social affairs, security, and resources. The second is the management index, focused on governance capacities in terms of steering capability and accountability. This examines the executive capacity of different actors to formulate, coordinate, and implement policies, as well as their accountability. The management index is a construct formed by the following variables: steering capability, policy implementation, institutional learning, and accountability. As with OECD data, the main limitation of Bertelsmann Stiftung indicators is the omission of Estonia and Slovenia (OECD members since 2010 but excluded from the Bertelsmann Stiftung study).

The framework also takes into account socio-cultural factors, as these are variables that affect how governments deal with addictions. To do so, we use the Inglehart's World Values Survey data (Inglehart and Welzel 2005, 2010), and the classification of the countries based on two major dimensions of cross-cultural variation: (1) traditional vs secular-rational and (2) survival vs self-expression values. The former reflects the contrast between societies in which religion is very important and those where it is not (World Values Survey 2012). On the other hand, survival/self-expression values are linked to the transition from an industrial society to a knowledge society, in which an increasing share of the population has grown up taking survival for granted. Their priorities have shifted from economic and physical security towards well-being, self-expression, and quality of life. World Values Survey data have been extracted from surveys conducted up to the year 2008. For those countries not covered in the 2008 wave survey, we have used data from a survey conducted between 1999 and 2004.

Table 2.1 presents how EU member states and Norway have been grouped according to all these indicators. All indicators affect and are correlated to the governance of addictions, but at the same time they have some limitations.

2.3 Information gathering for governance of addictions

The main documents compiled for each country were national strategies, action plans, legislation, and national evaluations. These documents provide a general approach to the directions and policy actions developed by the twenty-eight countries. Apart from these, we also reviewed specific documents focused on alcohol, tobacco, heroin, and cannabis. Regulation related to penalties for possessing, consuming, and trafficking illicit substances, as well as laws regulating production, distribution, age limits, advertising, and marketing of legal substances were also taken into account. We included national reports and documents produced by international organizations and agencies such as the World Health Organization (WHO), the United Nations (UN), and the European Monitoring Centre for Drugs and Drug Addictions (EMCDDA). This methodological approach is aligned with Quigley et al. (2013), who consider strategies, coordination systems, evaluation, public expenditure, and laws when analysing national policies on drugs.

With this information, our first step was to elaborate a holistic classification of public policies and programmes for addictions (see Figs 2.1 and 2.2). Until now, this classification was only available for specific substances. The points of departure for our literature review were Österberg and Karlsson (1998), the WHO Framework Convention on Tobacco Control (FCTC; WHO 2003), and

Table 2.1 Classification of countries according to contextual indicators

Country	Welfare state regime*	World Values Survey	OECD's Better Life Initiative**	Sustainable governance indicators**	Corruption Perception Index
Austria	Continental	n.a.	Material conditions	Moderate–high	Moderate–high
Belgium	Continental	Catholic Europe	Material conditions	Moderate	Moderate–high
Bulgaria	n.a.	Orthodox	n.a.	n.a.	Moderate–low
Cyprus	n.a.	n.a.	n.a.	n.a.	Moderate
Czech Rep.	n.a.	Catholic Europe	Standards	Moderate	Moderate–low
Denmark	Nordic	Protestant Europe	Quality of life	High	High
Estonia	n.a.	Ex-communist	Low performers	n.a.	Moderate
Finland	Nordic	Protestant Europe	Quality of life	High	High
France	Continental	Catholic Europe	Standards	Moderate	Moderate–high
Germany	Continental	Protestant Europe	Material conditions	Moderate–high	Moderate–high
Greece	Mediterranean	Catholic Europe	Low performers	Moderate–low	Moderate–low
Hungary	n.a.	Ex-communist	Low performers	Moderate	Moderate–low
Ireland	Anglo-Saxon	English-speaking	Quality of life	Moderate–high	Moderate–high
Italy	Mediterranean	Catholic Europe	Standards	Moderate	Moderate–low
Latvia	n.a.	Ex-communist	n.a.	n.a.	Moderate–low
Lithuania	n.a.	Catholic Europe	n.a.	n.a.	Moderate–low
Luxemburg	n.a.	Catholic Europe	Material conditions	Moderate–high	Moderate–high
Malta	n.a.	n.a.	n.a.	n.a.	Moderate

Netherlands	Nordic	Protestant Europe	Material conditions	Moderate-High	Moderate–high
Norway	Nordic	Protestant Europe	Quality of life	High	High
Poland	n.a.	Catholic Europe	Low performers	Moderate	Moderate
Portugal	Mediterranean	n.a.	Low performers	Moderate	Moderate
Romania	n.a.	Orthodox	n.a.	n.a.	Moderate–low
Slovakia	n.a.	Catholic Europe	Low performers	Moderate-Low	Moderate–low
Slovenia	n.a.	Catholic Europe	Standards	n.a.	Moderate
Spain	Mediterranean	Catholic Europe	Standards	Moderate	Moderate
Sweden	Nordic	Protestant Europe	Quality of life	High	High
UK	Anglo-Saxon	English-speaking	Material conditions	Moderate–high	Moderate–high

Notes: * Eastern European countries have not been classified since Esping-Andersen did not include them in his initial study. Nonetheless, a distinction can be introduced within the Central and East European countries (CEECs) according to Bohle and Greskovits (2006), with the Czech Republic, Hungary, Slovakia, and Slovenia on the one hand and, on the other, Estonia, Latvia, Lithuania, Bulgaria, and Romania.

** This is an OECD index; thus for non-OECD countries n.a. (not available) is stated.

Source: data from Esping-Andersen, G., *The three worlds of welfare capitalism*, Polity Press, Oxford, UK, Copyright © 1990; Ferrera, M., The 'Southern' model of welfare in social Europe', *Journal of European Social Policy*, Volume 6, Number1, pp. 17–37, Copyright © 1996 by SAGE Publications; *The Organisation for Economic Co-operation and Development (OECD), How's Life?: Measuring well-being*, OECD Publishing, Copyright © 2011 OECD; *Transparency International—Corruption Perception Index*, Copyright © 2011, available from www.cpi.transparency.org/cpi2012/; and *World Values Survey*, Copyright © 2012 World Values Survey, available from www.worldvaluessurvey.org.

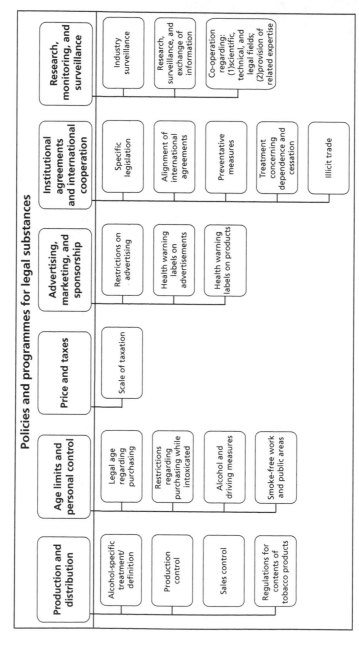

Fig. 2.1 Policies and programmes for legal substances

Source: data from Österberg, E. and Karlsson, T., *Alcohol policies in EU member states and Norway: A collection of country reports*, European Commission DG Health, Copyright © 1998; Joossens, L. and Raw, M., *The Tobacco Control Scale 2010 in Europe*, Association of the European Cancer Leagues, Belgium, Copyright © 2010; and from the authors' review of national strategies, action plans, evaluation documents.

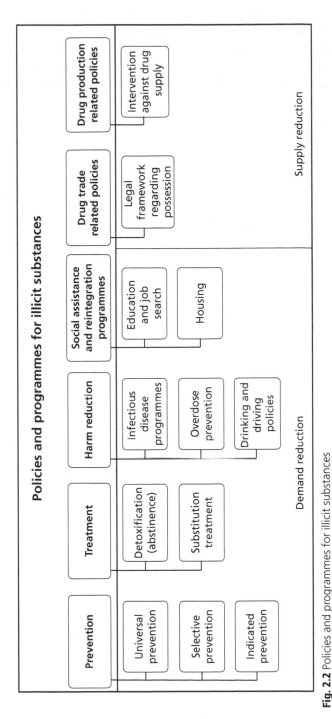

Fig. 2.2 Policies and programmes for illicit substances

Source: data from Babor, R., et al., Alcohol: *No Ordinary commodity: Research and public policy*, Oxford University Press, Oxford, UK, Copyright © 2010; Quigley, E., et al, *Illicit Drugs in Europe: Supply, demand and public policies*, Presentation at EMCDDA European Summer School, Copyright © 2013; and from the authors' review of national strategies, action plans, evaluation documents.

Joossens and Raw (2010) for legal substances, and Babor et al. (2010) and Quigley et al. (2013) on illicit substances. We also included in the classification the different policies we found during our empirical review of national strategies, action plans, and evaluation documents, for both legal and illicit substances.

For legal substances, public policies in Europe can be classified as follows: production and distribution; age limits and personal control; prices and taxes; advertising, marketing, and sponsorship; institutional agreements and international cooperation; research, monitoring, and surveillance. For the study of legal substances, more specifically for the analysis of alcohol policies, we took deeply into account the work conducted by Österberg and Karlsson (1998, 2003). This study provided us with sound data to analyse different countries and their policy performance in the field of alcohol. Specifically, the authors schematically present how each of the twenty-eight countries performs on the main alcohol policies, which are:

1 Alcohol definition

2 Control of production

3 Retail sale and distribution of alcoholic beverages

4 Age limits and personal control

5 Control of drunk driving

6 Control of advertising

7 Marketing and sponsorship of alcoholic beverages

8 Public policy and alcohol taxation and price.

Regarding tobacco, we use Joossens and Raw's (2010) Tobacco Control Scale, which quantifies the implementation of tobacco control policies at country level. Their scale aggregates seven policies (Joossens and Raw 2010):

1 Price increases through taxes on cigarettes and other tobacco products.

2 Bans and/or restrictions on smoking in public and work places.

3 Better consumer information, including public information campaigns and media.

4 Coverage and publicizing of research findings.

5 Comprehensive bans on the advertising and promotion of all tobacco products, including logos and brand names.

6 Large, direct health warning labels on cigarette boxes and other tobacco products.

7 Treatment to help dependent smokers stop, including increased access to medication.

Both scales, for alcohol and tobacco, are evidence-based policies recognized by researchers in the field of legal substances as appropriate measures to reduce the levels of consumption, prevent the misuse of these substances, and reduce the harm caused by heavy use over time.

For illicit substances the policies are: prevention; treatment; harm reduction; social assistance and reintegration programmes; drug trade related policies; and drug production related policies. These categories conform to a certain extent to the traditional demand and supply reduction classification; hence, we understand that this dichotomy is still very present in most of the countries analysed. Demand reduction involves policies and governmental actions aimed at reducing the desire of the citizens to consume legal and illicit addictive substances. On the other hand, supply reduction focuses attention on the manufacturing, distribution, and trafficking of illicit and legal addictive substances. Nonetheless, we avoided this taxonomy and focused on the six aforementioned policies, trying to reflect and highlight new trends that might lead to better and more effective policies.

Looking to the future, this methodological division between legal and illicit substances is unlikely to remain as consistent as it is now. Some countries, such as Denmark, are considering the legalization of cannabis (NordAN 2011), while others are pursuing a ban on tobacco consumption (for instance the Tobacco-Free Finland 2040 initiative). This is why, despite splitting them during the process of information gathering, we considered legal and illicit substances together to analyse the European governance of addictions.

2.4 Triangulation of sources of information

We took into account not only the content but also the whole political process of policy-making: how each country organizes its policy, which ministries and departments are involved along the planning, policy-making, and implementation process, and what kind of stakeholders, either public or private, are involved in the different stages of the governance of addictions. Furthermore, we also contrasted official information with that provided by national newspapers. Two national newspapers and a third economic newspaper were analysed for the twenty-eight countries. The newspapers were chosen based on their sales figures. We searched for news items about how governments and different stakeholders deal with one another and interact to define and implement addiction policies. The output of the media coverage was used to complement country tables and reports.

Furthermore, we conducted eighteen interviews with experts from fourteen EU countries. The interviewees were ALICE RAP participants, experts in the field of addiction focused on research (see Annex 1 for more information about the semi-structured interviews and interviewees). The interviews were in two parts, one on national issues and the other on the international domain. Finally, we sent a survey to national experts from around Europe with questions about their national policies on addiction, receiving ninety-one responses.

In summary, while focusing on the official governmental approach, we complemented and contrasted this with input from the media and experts, and introduced the main stakeholders involved in the policy-making and implementation processes. All this was complemented with an international perspective on the roles and impact of international organizations on addictions. Special emphasis was put on the role of the EU in governing addictions supranationally, and how it influences the policy-making of member states. It is worth noting that the EU has had a policy on drugs and addictions since the 1980s. However, member states still retain much of their sovereignty. Nevertheless, as shown in Chapter 3, the EU institutions have advanced towards harmonizing policies over the past three decades. The international analysis was complemented by the 'geopolitics of drugs', to help us understand why some countries are heavily impacted by international trafficking routes in their national policy-making. We considered the main trafficking routes, the effects of organized crime, and conflicts between lobbies and decision-makers.

We classified the data in country tables (see Annex 2 for the country table template). Firstly, the table presents contextual measures such as size, population, GDP, OECD Better Life Initiative, and progress. Secondly, it presents information on the country profile regarding addictions. This includes levels of consumption, international alignment with addiction-related treaties, and the geopolitical situation of the country in relation to drugs trafficking. Thirdly, the table contains information on national public policy on addictions, which includes the main focus of its current national strategy and action plan, but also looks at former strategies and action plans in order to map the political trend of the country. It also takes into consideration the ministries involved, the presence of an ad hoc organization to coordinate addiction policies, and the relation with businesses and non-profit organizations. Finally, a section on policy measures includes specific laws and regulations, how countries classify drugs according to the risks associated with them, and the penalties for possession, consumption, and drug trafficking. The table also includes good practices recognized by the EMCDDA and a policy timeline 2000–2011 in order to chart the evolution and whether election results affect policies on addiction. Using these country tables we prepared extensive country reports with in-depth data on contextual and policy measures plus all the information gathered through media coverage.

2.5 **Governance of addictions in Europe**

Therefore, the methodology we used was a comparative case analysis, using in-depth qualitative information and large N data. The bottom-up analysis—country by country—allowed us to analyse commonalities and differences in policy approaches. The final result from this process was the model to analyse the governance of addictions in Europe for this book (see Fig. 2.3).

The model builds on two levels of analysis: state factors and policy factors. Both levels are composed of a mix of quantitative and qualitative information. The state factors box includes indicators provided by welfare state regimes, the OECD Better Life Initiative, sustainable governance indicators, and the Corruption Perception Index. This level also embraces Inglehart's socio-cultural values, socio-economic indicators, the political structure of the country, and its interaction with the EU. On the other hand, the policy factors box focuses on how the country develops its policy on addictions. The country profile is a construct composed of a set of variables that affect the governance of addictions. The final output obtained from this analysis is the 'governance of addictions', which reflects how all these variables interrelate to develop the focus and organization of countries, and what kinds of strategy and structure are embedded in these countries to tackle drugs and addictions.

2.6 **European models of governance of addictions**

The qualitative study allowed us to present the main characteristics of each country. Next, we needed to be able quantitatively to analyse and compare whether there is one addictions model or several in Europe. For the quantitative analysis we used two traditional variables in management: strategy and structure. Strategy comprehends the focus and priorities of the policy; structure, on the other hand, encompasses the organizational and coordination systems developed to implement policy, as well as the involvement of public, businesses, and non-profit initiatives in the governance of addictions. The ends of the continuums are shown in Fig. 2.4.

At one end of the strategy axis is the safety and disease approach. This includes the characteristics shown by many countries, reflecting an approach that criminalizes the drug user, who is regarded as a psychiatrically diseased individual and/or an offender. Countries that implement this approach focus on supply reduction policies, heavily sanctioning the traffic and possession of illicit substances. This policy field is controlled by security-oriented ministries, such as the interior and justice ministries. The safety and disease approach translates into strict penalties and the absence of sophisticated distinctions of penalties depending on the risks associated with the substance.

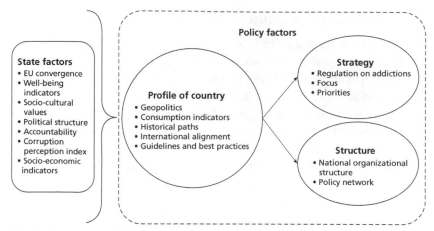

Fig. 2.3 Governance of addictions in Europe: model for the analysis

At the other end of the strategy continuum are the countries that take a well-being and relational management approach. Their policies are characterized by higher levels of social acceptance of substances and addictions. In these countries, citizens are in general more understanding about drug use and drug addicts because they take up the idea of individual freedom. This means that the focus here is on social consequences. The countries with a well-being and relational management approach tend to decriminalize the possession of drugs, implement harm reduction policies, and have evidence-based regulations. Hence, these countries decriminalize drug use and in some instances even drug possession in small quantities. They also embrace a social vision by taking into account the social consequences of substance consumption and substance addictions and dealing with them through harm reduction policies. Finally, the policies of most of these countries are evidence-based, and aimed at protecting the public and society in general through regulation.

The structure continuum focuses on the organizational structures that deal with addictions. At one end—substance-based reactive intervention—are the countries characterized by dividing policy structures in terms of substances and behaviours. They create new departments for any new addictive substance and behaviour. The advantage of this approach is high specialization; the disadvantage is a significant risk of lack of coordination. The countries at this end of the continuum tend to have little experience in the field, and policy inconsistencies arise from their lack of continuity regarding addictive substances. In this sense, they are considered followers of the EU guidelines, and their structures and policies aim to be aligned with those promoted by the EU. Furthermore, it

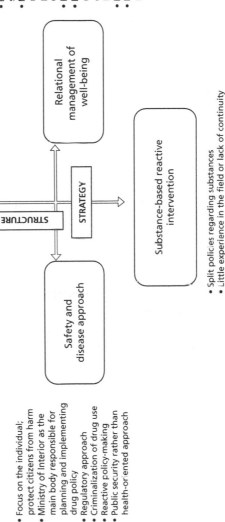

- Tackling of legal and illicit substances together
- Long experience in drug and addiction policies
- Complexity of organizational structures
- Multi-level governance and high levels of decentralization
- Involvement of stakeholders

Comprehensive policy: addictions and lifestyles

Relational management of well-being

- Focus on the public and society in general
- Ministry of Health as the main body responsible for planning and implementing drug policy
- Harm reduction approach
- Decriminalization of drug use: societal tolerance; ensure citizens' personal liberty
- Proactive policy making
- Health-oriented rather than public security approach

STRUCTURE

STRATEGY

- Focus on the individual; protect citizens from harm
- Ministry of Interior as the main body responsible for planning and implementing drug policy
- Regulatory approach
- Criminalization of drug use
- Reactive policy-making
- Public security rather than health-oriented approach

Safety and disease approach

Substance-based reactive intervention

- Split policies regarding substances
- Little experience in the field or lack of continuity
- Simplicity in organizational structures
- Centralized organizational structures
- Exclusion of stakeholders

Fig. 2.4 Strategy and structure in addictions policy

seems that policies and structures are only initiated when a problem appears; hence, they have reactive policy-making.

At the other end of the structure continuum are the countries with a comprehensive policy approach. They embrace holistic political strategies, including substances, either legal or illicit, and behaviours—addictions and lifestyles. Moreover, these countries tend to have extensive experience in drug and addiction policies, which normally leads to more complexity and the coordination of cross-cutting structures: more ministries, departments, and levels of government are involved and demonstrate higher levels of interdependence when dealing with drug-related problems.

2.7 Cluster analysis of addiction policies in Europe

The process by which we group the twenty-eight countries is based on nineteen indicators, ten for strategy and nine for structure. In Fig. 2.5 the operationalization of the variables for the cluster analysis are introduced (see Annex 3 for an in-depth explanation of each of the measures).

With those measures we have clustered the approaches for the twenty-eight countries (see Fig. 2.6). Cluster analysis is an exploratory tool, not an inferential one. It is aimed at identifying groups within data that share similar features but are also different from other groups. We have a matrix with C countries and I items, or indicators, that represent characteristics of the policies. The CxI matrix is used to guess which countries tend to have similar policies, and its transpose IxC is used to guess which policies tend to go together.

More specifically, we use Gower's similarity measure, which takes into account symmetric combinations. Symmetric combinations are convenient since we give the same importance to the fact of having a characteristic as not having it. We are interested in pure bi-directional similarity, not in the similarity of having characteristics only. This means that having or not having a policy is equally important for calculating the distances between countries. Once similarity measures between countries and policy items are produced, the distances between them are organized using hierarchical clustering. Hierarchical clustering implies that the data themselves choose the number of clusters. This contrasts with traditional cluster analysis, where the researcher imposes the number of clusters. More specifically, we employ the Ward method of agglomeration, which minimizes the sum of the squares of the distances.

The map with the final results is shown in Fig. 2.7 and explained in-depth in the following chapters.

Strategy

1. Ministry of Health
Is the Ministry of Health responsible for drug and addiction policies?
(Y = 1 | N = 0)

2. Classification determines penalties
Does drug classification determine penalties? (Y = 1 | N = 0)

3. Decriminalize possession
Does the country embrace decriminalization policies? (Y = 1 | N = 0)

4. Injection rooms
Does the country provide injection rooms? (Y = 1 | N = 0) proxy for harm reduction

5. Alcohol policy scales
Does the country rank above the EU average in the alcohol policy scale?
(Y = 1 | N = 0)

6. Tobacco control scale
Does the country rank above the EU average in the tobacco control scale?
(Y = 1 | N = 0)

7. Supply reduction in national strategy
Supply reduction is not one of the priorities in the National strategy of
the country. (Y = 1 | N = 0)
Versus treatment, prevention and harm reduction

8. Public health in national strategy
Does the national strategy have a public-health perspective on
its aims? (Y = 1 | N = 0)

9. Well-being in national strategy
Does the national strategy has a well-being perspective on its aims?
(Y = 1 | N = 0)

10. Best practices
Has been the country recognized for having the highest degree (3 out of 1,2,3) of
EMCDDA best practices? (Y = 1 | N = 0)

Structure

1. Tackle legal and illicit substances together
Does the country tackle together licit and illicit substances? (Y = 1 | N = 0)

2. Transversality
Ratio of ministries involved in the governance of drugs and addictions
(>50% = 1 | <50% = 0)

3. Nonprofit organizations in decision-making
Are non-profit organizations involved in the decision-making process? (Y = 1 | N = 0)

4. Private organizations in decision-making
Are private organizations involved in the decision-making process? (Y = 1 | N = 0)

5. Ad hoc coordinator body
Has the country a coordinator or an ad hoc body for addictions? (Y = 1 | N = 0)

6. Policy making devolution
Does this country devolve policy-making to decentralized structures? (Y = 1 | N = 0)

7. Implementation devolution
Does this country devolve implementation to decentralized structures?
(Y = 1 | N = 0)

8. Addiction on objectives
Is the concept of addiction on the objectives of the national strategy?
(Y = 1 | N = 0)

9. Trajectory
Has this country long standing regulatory policies on drugs?
(Before the 1st EU report = 1 | After the 1st EU report = 0)

Fig. 2.5 Operationalization of variables for the cluster analysis

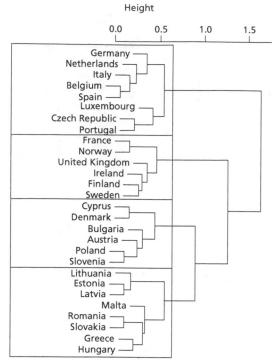

Fig. 2.6 Results for the cluster analysis of addictions in Europe

2.8 **Challenges and limitations of the research**

This is the first time that this kind of study, aimed at determining the models of governance of addictions in the EU, has been conducted, which makes it both a challenge and an opportunity. The book looks at the strategic picture of how the twenty-eight countries develop their governance of addictions. Thus, when grouping the countries, the emphasis is placed on the strategy of each country and its organizational design without losing sight of the theoretical framework and contextual variables. The following chapters not only present the different models but also describe each country's governance of addictions and justify why it has been grouped in each model.

There are some limitations to our methodology. The first is insufficient information to provide a complete view of relational governance. We have solved this, as much as possible, by using media coverage, expert interviews, and a survey. Second, the accessibility and language of official documents has hindered the analysis and slowed down the work process, since it has been

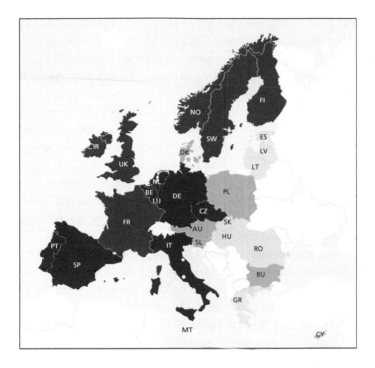

Model 1: Trendsetters in illicit substances

Model 2: Regulators of legal substances

Model 3: Transitioning model

Model 4: Traditional approach

AU	Austria	FI	Finland	LV	Latvia	PT	Portugal
BE	Belgium	FR	France	LT	Lithuania	RO	Romania
BU	Bulgaria	DE	Germany	LU	Luxemburg	SK	Slovakia
CY	Cyprus	GR	Greece	MT	Malta	SL	Slovenia
CZ	Czech Republic	HU	Hungary	NL	Netherlands	SP	Spain
DK	Denmark	IR	Ireland	NO	Norway	SW	Sweden
ES	Estonia	IT	Italy	PL	Poland	UK	United Kingdom

* These abbreviations for the countries are used for the figures throughout this book.

Fig. 2.7 Models of governance of addictions in Europe

necessary to translate some documents. Third, not all contextual frameworks that are used cover the twenty-eight countries. We tackled this limitation through the construction of a compendium of other contextual and control variables. Fourth, it could be claimed that we only focus on the national level and that federal states, regions, and cities can have relevant policies that in some aspects can be directly contradictory of each other. That being so, we have to state that our intention is to provide an overview at the EU level to identify the starting point from which the governance of addictions needs to be redesigned. This does not allow us to dwell on specific policies provided by regions and local governments, although we do recognize their relevance.

Fifth, this book deals with only four substances, heroin, cannabis, tobacco, and alcohol. We consider that these four substances provide a broad picture of how the twenty-eight countries are tackling addictions and drug abuse. Future research should tackle other relevant substances, such as cocaine and synthetic drugs, and take into account behavioural addictions such as gambling. Although this will be the focus of the ALICE RAP series, when relevant, other substances and even addictive behaviours have been taken into account in order to understand better the governance model of a country.

Furthermore, it is noteworthy that the classification is continuous and dynamic, and the classification of each country can vary over time. More interestingly, this first attempt to present governance of addictions regimes can also be used to compare the twenty-eight countries analysed with other non-European countries, allowing us to see how far the latter differ from the four approaches we present or whether they are aligned with any of the four clusters presented.

Despite all these limitations, this work is an opportunity and a point of departure for future studies in the field of governance and addictions. The establishment of different models allows experts in the field to analyse new and better ways to deal with addictions and redesign their governance approach. Within the ALICE RAP project, this book is conceived as a cornerstone on which to build the future perspective of how addictions can be tackled.

Chapter 3

European Union achievements and the role of international organizations

3.1 Introduction to EU policy on addictions

Before presenting each of the models generated by the cluster analysis, we begin by describing the processes by which the EU policy on addictions has been established and institutionalized. We also analyse to what extent the EU influences the governance of addictions at member-state level and the resulting typologies. We examine the features of the governance of addictions and the ground on which is has built up in the EU over the last three decades. Two main matters have to be taken into account: the broader context and geopolitical developments, such as the trafficking flows in Europe; and the leading and coordination role hold by international organizations—particularly the UN and the WHO—whose policy orientations, reports, and resolutions have influenced the development of EU policy.

3.2 The EU addiction policy process: A historical perspective

Although the EU was founded in 1958 with the Treaty of Rome establishing the European Economic Community (EEC), it was not until the 1980s that the EU began to take drug issues seriously (see Table 3.1). The reasons for this lack of attention to the subject during these years include, among others, the fact that the EEC was eminently an economic instrument, thus not focusing that much on social issues, the leading role of WHO and UNODC (United Nations Office on Drugs and Crime), and that it was not until the 1980s that the alarm was raised over the heroin crisis and the HIV epidemic.

The EU as a whole began grappling with illicit and legal drugs and the associated problems in the second half of the 1980s—a decade that saw on one side a boom in heroin and cocaine use and growing awareness of HIV/AIDS, and on the other a demand for the harmonization of several commercial matters related to legal drugs (commercialization, marketing, and advertising).

Table 3.1 Key EU activities on drugs

Year	Key EU activity on drugs
1988	Participation in the Conference on the illicit traffic in narcotic drugs and psychotropic substances, Vienna.
1988	Ratification of the UN Convention against illicit traffic in narcotic drugs and psychotropic substances.
1988	Creation at the initiative of the European Parliament of a specific line in the European budget to combat drugs.
1989	Creation of the European Committee to Combat Drugs (CELAD) composed of the national drug coordinators of the EEC member states.
1990	Adoption by the Rome European Council of the first European plan to combat drugs.
1992	Signing of the Maastricht Treaty on European Union, which refers for the first time in an EU Treaty to the fight against drugs within the public-health framework.
1992	Revision of the first European plan to combat drugs approved by the Edinburgh European Council in December.
1993	Entry into force of the Maastricht Treaty on European Union.
1994	Creation of the Europol Drugs Unit, the forerunner to Europol, as a non-operational unit.
1995	Conference on 'Policies towards drugs in Europe', jointly organized by the European Parliament, the Presidency of the EU Council of Ministers and the European Commission, March.
1995	Adoption of a new EU Action Plan to combat drugs, 1995–1999.
1996	Adoption of the Community action programme on the prevention of drug dependence, 1996–2000.
1998	Entry into force of the Europol Convention.
1999	Comprehensive action plan on drugs (EU–Latin America).
1999	Entry into force on 1 May of the Treaty of Amsterdam strengthening the provisions on drugs included in the Maastricht Treaty.
1999	Adoption by the European Council of the European Union drugs strategy (2000–2004).
2000	Endorsement of the EU action plan on drugs (2000–2004).
2001	Adoption by the Commission of the Communication to the Council and the European Parliament on the implementation of the EU action plan on drugs (2000–2004).
2002	EU Action Plan on Drugs between the EU and the Central Asian Republics.
2002	Adoption by the Commission of the Communication to the Council and the European Parliament on the mid-term evaluation of the EU action plan on drugs (2000–2004).

Table 3.1 (continued) Key EU activities on drugs

Year	Key EU activity on drugs
2002	Adoption of a new community action programme for public health.
2003	EU Action Plan on Drugs between the EU and the Western Balkans.
2004	Adoption of the EU drugs strategy (2005–2012).
2005	Endorsement by the Commission of a Communication on a EU Drugs Action Plan (2005–2008).
2005	Endorsement by the Council of the EU Drugs Action Plan (2005–2008).
2006	EU Alcohol Strategy (2006–2012).
2006	EU Action Plan on Drugs between the EU and Afghanistan.
2006	EU Action plan on Drugs between the EU and Russia.
2006	Green paper on the Role of Civil Society in Drugs Policy in Europe.
2006	Recast of the regulation creating the EMCDDA.
2007	Report from the Commission on the implementation of the Council Recommendation of 18 June 2003 on the prevention and reduction of health-related harm associated with drug dependence.
2007	Adoption by the European Parliament and the Council of the specific programme Drug Prevention and Information 2007–2013 as part of the general programme Fundamental Rights and Justice.
2008	Council adopts a decision defining BZP as a new psychoactive substance that is to be made subject to control measures and criminal provisions.
2008	Report of the final evaluation of the EU Drugs Action Plan (2005–2008).
2008	Endorsement by the Council of the EU Drugs Action Plan (2009–12).
2009	Entry into force of the Lisbon Treaty.
2009	EU Action Plan on Drugs between the EU and the Central Asian States.
2009	EU Action Plan on Drugs between the EU and the Western Balkans (2009–2013).
2011	Adoption of the Action Plan to fight smuggling of cigarettes and alcohol along the EU Eastern border.
2013	Entry into force of the new EU drugs strategy (2013–2020).
2013	Adoption of the EU Action Plan on Drugs (2013–2016).

First, in 1982 the European Parliament drew up a report on combating drug abuse. Three years later, the European Parliament set up the Stewart-Clark Committee (we thank Sir Jack Stewart-Clark, who was interviewed for the benefit of this chapter) to investigate drug problems in EU member states. The aim of the Committee was to learn about the problem and bring influence to bear on the Council and the European Commission to increase awareness and take action on the basis of its findings and recommendations. Unanimous agreement eluded the Committee, given the rift between members advocating a law enforcement approach and those favouring health-oriented and harm-reduction policies (Elvins 2003). The report was finally submitted in 1986 and presented recommendations aimed at increasing prevention and education measures and boosting international cooperation to combat drug trafficking. Furthermore, the document introduced supply and demand reduction recommendations and was accompanied by a statement of the minority position, which supported a range of health-oriented policies (Bewley-Taylor 2012).

The EU Council passed a resolution in the same year, based upon the Stewart-Clark Committee report. It aligned with the Single Convention on Narcotic Drugs (UN 1961) as amended by the 1972 Protocol and the Convention on Psychotropic Substances (UN 1971a). Both the Convention and the Protocol focused on drugs from the criminal law standpoint. Despite being in a minority, health-oriented supporters on the Stewart-Clark Committee succeeded in introducing a more liberal approach to cannabis use. Even so, the Council opted for the UN Convention's approach.

The vision of the Stewart-Clark report can also be seen in the establishment of the Trevi Group, a body investigating organized crime and drug trafficking at the strategic, tactical, and technical levels (Bunyan 1993). The Trevi Group gathers together ministers of the interior and justice from the EEC. On 1985 at a Trevi ministers' meeting in Rome, the role of Trevi 3 was redefined to look at organized crime and drug trafficking at the strategic, tactical, and technical levels. The influence of the Trevi Group, together with the Schengen Agreement of 1985, promoted the dominance of supply-side measures and a law enforcement oriented approach (Bewley-Taylor 2012). The relevance of Schengen is particularly notable in relation to drug trafficking, due to the dismantling of internal European border controls. This was one of the main reasons why the EU started to encourage cooperation between member states. It also explains why cooperation in combating trafficking and organized crime is currently one of the most highly developed areas of the EU's drugs policy.

In 1988 the EEC (later to morph into the EU) signed Article 12.2 of the UN Convention against illicit traffic in narcotic drugs and psychotropic substances

(UN 1988). This was the first time that the EU had taken part in a UN drugs conference for nation states. The 1980s ended with the establishment of CELAD (European Committee to Combat Drugs) in 1989, which took up the Stewart-Clark report recommendations. This ad hoc political group brought together representatives from EU member states and examined social and health aspects of the drug problem in Europe, as well as drug trafficking and penal sanctions.

EU policies and regulation on legal drugs (tobacco and alcohol) also started by the end of the 1980s. The 1989 Council directive on television broadcasting established that 'all forms of television advertising for cigarettes and other tobacco products shall be prohibited' (Article 13). Furthermore, Article 15 defined the criteria for the televised advertising of alcoholic drinks, focusing specially on protecting minors. It also forbad any link between alcohol consumption and driving, or enhancing physical performance, prohibited the creation of any impression that the consumption of alcohol contributes to social or sexual success, and stated that advertising should neither encourage immoderate consumption of alcohol nor present abstinence or moderation in a negative light. Also in 1989, the Council adopted a resolution on banning smoking in places open to the public. This resolution ensured that in case of conflict, the right to health of non-smokers prevailed over the right of smokers to smoke.

The establishment of CELAD was a significant step in institutionalizing an EU policy on drugs. Its work drew strongly on the first European Plan to Combat Drugs adopted by the EU's Council of Ministers held in Rome in December 1990 (Van Solinge 1999). This plan sought to draw up a coherent action against drugs at the EU level and focused on demand-reduction policies, measures to combat illicit trafficking, and greater coordination at member-state level. This EU action plan (and all subsequent EU action plans) focused solely on illicit substances and did not include legal drugs such as alcohol and tobacco. The formalization of an EU drug policy took a stride with the inclusion of drugs in the Maastricht Treaty of 1993. Also in 1993, the EU established the EMCDDA (Council of the European Communities 1993), which began work a year later. The Europol Drugs Unit (EDU) became operational in 1994.

At the beginning of the 1990s the European Parliament (EP) published the Cooney Report (1992) on the effects of drug trafficking and organized crime. This report stressed the importance of demand- and harm-reduction policies and the need for governments to spend more on reducing the risks of drug use. The report also 'recommended that the possession of drugs for personal use should no longer be considered a criminal offence' (Van Solinge 2002: 59). The Cooney Report proved unable to rally support from EU institutions and was never officially adopted.

In 1995 the EU approved its third action (see Fig. 3.1) to promote greater cooperation among member states with a view to reducing both drug supply and demand in the EU. It was drawn up by national drugs experts (a precursor to what later became the Horizontal Drugs Group, or HDG). The experts devised recommendations that were incorporated into the Community Action Programme on the Prevention of Drug Dependence (1996–2000). It provided a comprehensive framework and a common EU approach in three areas: demand reduction, the fight against drugs trafficking, and action at the international level.

The institutionalization of the EU drug policy was completed in the late 1990s and came through EU participation and influence over the 1988 Special Session of the UN General Assembly (UNGASS) to deliberate on the global drugs problem. In that session, the 'EU emphasis on demand reduction gained ground in relation to the American law enforcement approach that had been more traditional in UN circles' (Van Solinge 2002: 15). Another milestone was the strengthening of the Maastricht provisions on drugs in the Amsterdam Treaty of 1999.

At the organizational level, in 1997 the Committee of Permanent Representatives (COREPER) set up the HDG—a cross-cutting body that played a coordinating role in all drug-related issues. This group prepared all relevant legislation and political documents adopted by the Council. It also monitored and chased up drug-related activities in all EU bodies, preventing duplication of work, highlighting gaps, and suggesting new initiatives. However, the fact that health-related policies were mainly the responsibility of member states led the EU to focus most on law enforcement, police control policies, and international cooperation.

A Council Directive 92/84 (Council of the European Communities 1992a) on the approximation of the rates of excise duty on alcohol and alcoholic beverages established that, from 1993, the minimum rate of excise duty on wine (still and sparkling) was fixed at European Currency Unit (ECU) 0 per hectolitre of product. The entrance of Finland and Sweden into the EU (1995) had a profound impact on EU alcohol policies. During the Finnish presidency in 1999, the Council discussed the need to address the issue of alcohol and young people (Ugland 2011).

In contrast to alcohol, which had not had any Council directive, regulation, or recommendation during the 1990s, the Council passed one regulation on the common organization of the market in raw tobacco 2075/92 (Council of the European Communities 1992b) and one directive on the introduction of measures to encourage improvements in the safety and health at work of pregnant workers and workers who have recently given birth or are breastfeeding (Council

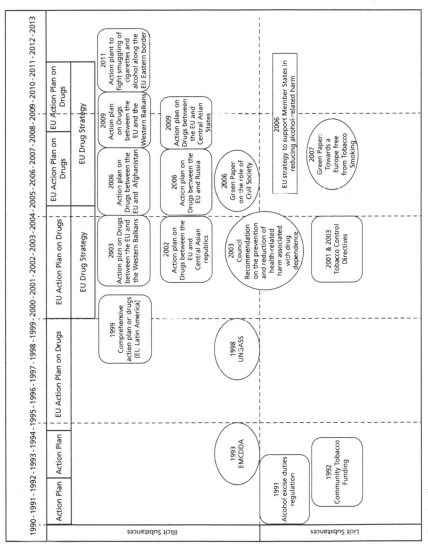

Fig. 3.1 EU drug policy timeline

of the European Communities 1992c). Furthermore, in 2007 the Council of the EU (2007) passed a second directive amending and updating the Council Directive 89/552/EEC concerning the pursuit of television broadcasting activities. In 1996 the Council passed a resolution on the reduction of smoking in the European Community (Council of the EU 1996) with the purpose of contributing to a review of existing and possible future anti-smoking strategies both at community and member-state levels.

During 1999 the policy on drugs and addictions at EU level was strengthened by the Amsterdam Treaty and the Tampere Summit, which underlined the need for a comprehensive approach to the drugs problem. In 2000 the EU approved its first strategy on drugs, focusing on reducing supply and demand and introducing international cooperation as one of its pillars. This first EU strategy on drugs represented a shift towards health-oriented policies. The EU thus began to give harm reduction and public health greater emphasis. The Treaty of Amsterdam gave new scope for health protection, drug control, and police and judicial cooperation. It also envisaged establishing common rules for tackling organized crime, terrorism, and drug trafficking.

In 2003 the European Council of Ministers approved a recommendation on 'the prevention and reduction of health-related harm associated with drug dependence' (Council of the EU 2003b). A year later, at the 47th Commission on Narcotic Drugs (CND), the central policy-making body within the UN system dealing with drug-related matters, the EU made a broadly supportive statement on harm reduction despite fierce opposition from the Swedes (Bewley-Taylor 2012). Swedish discomfort at introducing harm reduction in public documents reappeared at the high-level summit at CND's 2009 meeting, which showed how internal rifts could cripple the EU in the field of drug control.

The second EU drugs strategy was eight years in the making and was the framework for developing two action plans, the first running from 2005 to 2008 and the second from 2009 to 2012. The strategy aims to 'protect and improve the well-being of society and of the individual, to protect public health, to offer a high level of security for the general public and to take a balanced, integrated approach to the drugs problem' (Council of the EU 2004a: 2). The most outstanding feature of these strategies and action plans was their focus on reducing both supply and demand. Furthermore, the EU also introduced two cross-cutting issues: (1) greater cooperation at both EU and international levels; (2) research, information, and evaluation.

This strategy faces drugs as a cross-cutting problem that requires the involvement of welfare, health, education, justice, and home affairs as well as international collaboration with non-EU states. For the first time, this strategy and both action plans included the term 'harm reduction' within the 'demand reduction' section. This new trend towards more health-oriented strategies and action plans covering harm-reduction policies stemmed partly from the Dutch presidency of HDG. Following the Council Recommendations of 2003, the Dutch 'pushed for the explicit inclusion of the term harm reduction within the EU Strategy' (Bewley-Taylor 2012: 89).

In 2001 and 2003, an EP and Council approved two tobacco product directives (Council of the EU 2001, 2003a). These laid the groundwork to approximate the laws, regulations, and administrative provisions of member states concerning the advertising and sponsorship of tobacco products, the maximum tar, nicotine, and carbon monoxide yields of cigarettes, and the health warnings and other information to appear on unit packets of tobacco products. These are the two basic laws upon which the EU based its tobacco control policy, which was complemented by directives on the structure and rates of excise duty applied on manufactured tobacco and the work of OLAF (the European Anti-Fraud Office), which focused on illicit tobacco trading. However, EU ambitions to reduce tobacco consumption went beyond that and in 2007 the EC released a green paper, 'Towards a Europe free from tobacco smoke: policy options at EU level' (EC 2007a).

In 2010 the EC launched a public consultation to interested stakeholders in order to revise the tobacco product directive. The aim of this revision was to improve awareness of the dangers of tobacco use, increase motivation to quit, and discourage the initiation of smoking. The final product of this consultation was a proposal for a directive passed in 2012 (EC 2012), to come into force in 2014. In this directive the European Commission adopted a rule that reserves up to 60 per cent of the packaging to include deterrent images and text, and prohibited any smell or taste (e.g. menthol) that camouflages the characteristics of cigarettes (Abellán 2012).

Comparing its alcohol and tobacco policies, the EU has been able to establish a control policy on tobacco, in line with and complementary to the WHO Tobacco Convention Framework ratified by all EU member states, which is legally binding for member states; however, it has been unable to pass binding regulations or directives for alcohol. On the other hand, alcohol and illicit drug strategies and action plans have to be considered as recommendations that can be followed by member states. In this respect, the Alcohol Strategy of 2006 can be interpreted as a success, but there are no means to enforce it, as it is a Council conclusion. In addition, regardless of some attempts to rule on minimum taxes, alcohol taxation is still at the discretion of member states (subsidiary principle). What's more, national alcohol polices have been indirectly affected by EU policies due to the Schengen Agreement and free trade between member states. In this context, the current trend towards decriminalization of some illicit drugs (cannabis) should be analysed, bearing in mind the difficulties in building public-health policies around legal substances (alcohol) in a free trade paradigm.

3.3 **Stakeholder involvement in EU policy-making on addictions**

There is a well-known wish to involve civil society in EU policy-making and implementation. This can be seen in the EU Action Plan 2009–12, which states: 'It is time to put the people of Europe at the centre of policy in this field and to get Europe's citizens more involved.' (Council of the EU 2008: 2). As a first step, the Commission helped set up the European Civil Society Forum on Drugs in 2006.

Despite the EU's wish to take civil society views into account, the main players implementing measures are the Council of Ministers, the Commission, member states, the Presidency, EMCDDA, Europol, Eurojust, EMA, and the UN through the Dublin Group (see Fig. 3.2). The Dublin Group is a flexible, informal consultation and coordination mechanism for global, regional, and country-specific problems of illicit drugs production, trafficking, and demand. Its members are the twenty-seven EU member states plus Australia, Canada, Japan, Norway, the USA, the European Commission, and the UNODC. Civil

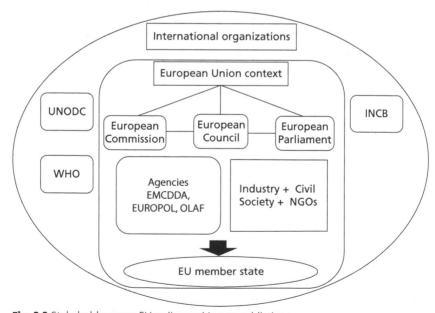

Fig. 3.2 Stakeholder map: EU policy-making on addictions

society groups and their umbrella associations at EU level are not yet involved in implementing action plans but those NGO networks represented in the Civil Society Forum do take part in the evaluation of action plans.

On the companies' side, the main stakeholders are the alcohol and tobacco industries and foundations. The alcohol industry has three main lobbies at EU level: SpiritsEUROPE, which embraces the European Forum for Responsible Drinking (EFRD), previously known as the Amsterdam Group; the Brewers of Europe (BoE); and the Comité Européen des Entreprises Vins (CEEV). These associations work in different domains, influencing especially policies related to the international market, external trade, spirits, and society, taxation, and the environment. Both SpiritsEUROPE and BoE act as pressure groups mainly to the EC. EFRD is an alliance of Europe's leading spirits companies. It supports the targeting of specific drinking problems but believes that this issue should be kept separate from alcohol consumption in general. It maintains that most people drink responsibly and without harmful consequences.

Apart from the four leading tobacco companies (Altria/Philip Morris; Japan Tobacco; British American Tobacco; and Imperial Tobacco), the tobacco industry has four associations that bring together these companies with other interested private stakeholders and national manufacturers' associations: the Confederation of European Community Cigarette Manufacturers (CECCM), the European Cigar Manufacturers Association (ECMA), the European Smoking Tobacco Association (ESTA), and the European Confederation of Tobacco Retailers (ECTR). These associations aim to influence and promote ongoing dialogue with EU institutions and participate constructively in the EU decision-making process.

On the civil society side there are also organizations that review the initiatives for each substance and look at cross-cutting initiatives. Examples presented in this chapter include the European Civil Society Forum on Drugs (CSF), the European Public Health Alliance (EPHA), and the European Alcohol Policy Alliance. The CSF is a product of a 2006 green paper on the Role of Civil Society in Drugs Policy in the European Union, the aim of which was to create a 'practical instrument to support policy formulation and implementation through practical advice' (EC 2006b: 8). Since 2011, this forum has brought together thirty-five organizations[1] once a year and serves as a talking shop for the Commission and civil society organizations. The three main aims of the CSF are to feed specific grass-roots experience into Commission proposals, contribute to the work on monitoring the EU Drugs Action Plan, and support the EC's work in preparing a new EU drugs policy framework.

Another civil society group, this time focusing on reducing the harm done by the consumption of tobacco and alcohol, is the European Public Health Alliance

(EPHA). EPHA is a non-profit organization for fostering better health registered in Belgium. There are also pressure groups covering specific substances, such as EUROCARE and EURAD. The European Alcohol Policy Alliance is an alliance of around fifty-five non-governmental public health and social organizations from twenty-three countries in Europe; it has been working on the prevention and reduction of alcohol-related harm in Europe since 1990. Europe Against Drugs is a non-profit organization devoted to advocating a prevention- and recovery-oriented drug policy at national and international levels.

As an example of the participation process that the EU would like to make available to civil society and the industry, in 2007 the EC launched the so-called European Alcohol and Health Forum (a civil society forum). This forum, which has over forty members, forms a cornerstone of the implementation of the 2006 Alcohol Strategy. The overall objective is to provide a common platform for all interested stakeholders at EU level who pledge to step up actions relevant to reducing alcohol-related harm (EC 2007b).

Research institutes, centres, and universities also play a relevant role by providing evidence of the health and social costs of legal and illicit drugs and evidence-based policy proposals. They have a direct influence when they are asked to join meetings, task forces, or science groups as experts or to produce technical and background reports on topics to be discussed later among the EU institutions. One of these is RAND Europe, an independent non-profit research institute whose mission is to help improve policy and decision-making through research and analysis, which has assessed, among others, the tobacco products directive (Tiessen et al. 2010). Other relevant institutions are Trimbos Instituut, the Institut für Therapieforschung München, the Zeus Gmbh Centre for Applied Psychology, Social and Environmental Research, the IVO Addiction Research Institute Foundation, the IDT Institute on Drugs and Drug Addiction, and the UTRIP Institute for Research and Development.

3.4 Impact of addictive substances and geopolitics in European regions and countries

In order to gain a global understanding of the different drug-related problems in Europe, and how European regions and countries are affected by different addictive substances, we examined the impact and geopolitics of the four substances (heroin, cannabis, tobacco, and alcohol).

3.4.1 The geopolitics of heroin

Heroin still accounts for the greatest share of morbidity and mortality from drug abuse in the EU (EMCDDA 2011a). According to the UNODC 2011 Drug

Report, Afghanistan remains the world's largest illicit opium-producing country, accounting for 74 per cent of global opium production in 2010. The heroin produced in Afghanistan reaches the EU through two main routes: the Balkan Route and the Silk Road. The former has its roots in Turkey, which is a major staging area and transportation route for heroin for European markets (UNODC 2011a).

On the EU side, the most badly affected member states for heroin are Bulgaria and Greece. Both countries are the gateway to the EU for traffickers smuggling heroin (EMCDDA 2011b). Most of the heroin bound for the western and central European consumer markets is transported overland to the Netherlands and, to a lesser degree, Belgium (EMCDDA 2008a). Other EU countries with high levels of heroin seizures are the UK, France, and Italy (EMCDDA 2010). These nations are the target markets, whereas Bulgaria, for example, is a staging post.

Reducing the supply of heroin to the EU means fostering stability in Afghanistan and, at the same time, fostering greater police cooperation between Turkey and the EU. Between 2002 and 2006 the EC contributed €250 million to develop sustainable alternatives to poppy cultivation for farmers in north and northeast Afghanistan (EMCDDA 2008a).

3.4.2 The geopolitics of cannabis

As UNODC authors state, estimating cannabis traffic is even harder than for heroin because of the sheer number of places where cannabis is grown and the trend for consumers to 'grow their own' (EMCDDA 2008b: 187). While many cannabis plants are grown in EU countries, cannabis resin is mainly produced in Morocco and exported to the EU. Cannabis is thus the most heavily consumed illicit substance in the EU. It is estimated that 22.5 per cent of EU adults have used the drug at least once (Council of the EU 2011). Spain occupies a strategic geographical position as it represents one of the main European gateways for cannabis trafficking from Morocco (it reports the largest cannabis resin seizures worldwide).

In terms of the EU policy on cannabis, apart from the Framework Decision (Council of the EU 2004b), which recommends penalties for consumption, possession, and trafficking of illicit substances, there is only one Council Resolution on cannabis, which was passed in 2004 (Council of the EU 2004c). The resolution requests member states to take measures to discourage personal use of cannabis, such as enhancing communication with cannabis users, especially the very young; informing and training parents, teachers, media professionals, prison staff, and police officers; and promoting networking among health and education professionals on cannabis-related issues. The Council also invites member states to take measures against internet sites providing information on the cultivation and promotion of cannabis.

3.4.3 Tobacco

With more than 650,000 tobacco-related deaths a year—a figure that represents more than 15 per cent of all EU deaths—smoking remains one of the largest avoidable causes of morbidity and premature death in the EU (Tiessen et al. 2010). Since the 1980s, the prevalence of smoking has been declining; in 2012, on average, 29 per cent of the EU populations smoked, and the EU mean of the number of cigarettes smoked cigarettes per day was 14.4. One should note that no fewer than thirteen EU member states produce tobacco; regions in Italy, Greece, Spain, and Bulgaria are particularly active. Moreover, the EU is the world's biggest tobacco importer (EC-DG Agriculture and Rural Development 2012).

Although the EU has no specific strategies or action plans on tobacco, as a result of internal market regulations, the EC has produced two directives (one on tobacco control and another on tobacco advertising) and two Council recommendations on preventing smoking and on smoke-free areas. It has also launched many projects to raise awareness of the health hazards of smoking and to reduce the number of people who start smoking. One of the main policies in this respect is the directive on the structure and rates of excise duty applied on manufactured tobacco, which 'shall represent at least 57 per cent of the weighted average retail selling price of cigarettes released for consumption' (Council of the EU 2010a: 2). Tobacco smuggling is also on the EU agenda, as seen in its 2011 'Action plan to fight against smuggling of cigarettes and alcohol along the EU eastern border'.

Private tobacco companies play an active role in implementing policies, especially through agreements for combating smuggling. It is worth noting that contraband, counterfeit, and smuggled tobacco causes large losses in the EU member states' tax revenues. Specifically, the EC and OLAF have signed agreements with the main businesses manufacturing and producing cigarettes: Altria/Philip Morris (2004)—main tobacco products are L&M, Marlboro, Parliament, Red & White; Japan Tobacco (2007)—main products are Camel and Winston; British American Tobacco (2010)—main products are Kent, Lucky Strike, and Pall Mall; and Imperial Tobacco (2010)—main products are Ducados and Fortuna. These agreements aim to work with member states' law enforcement authorities to fight against the counterfeiting and smuggling of cigarettes.

3.4.4 **Alcohol**

The EU per capita alcohol consumption is over twice the world average (Amphora 2012). Alcohol abuse is the cause of 12.5 per cent of the deaths of those aged between 15 and 64. The EU is the largest exporter of spirit drinks in the world (2011), worth €8.5 billion. In contrast with its strategies on heroin, cannabis, and tobacco, the EU has a specific strategy on alcohol. The EU Alcohol Strategy was approved in 2006 and ran to the end of 2012. Two years before its approval, the EC held extensive consultations with member states' experts, international organizations, researchers, and stakeholders, taking into account differing views and positions.

The strategy, which supports member states in mitigating alcohol-related harm, establishes five priorities for EU measures on alcohol consumption: to (1) protect young people, children, and unborn children; (2) reduce injuries and deaths from alcohol-related road traffic accidents; (3) prevent alcohol-related harm among adults and reduce the negative impact in the workplace; (4) inform, educate, and raise awareness on the impact of harmful and hazardous alcohol consumption, and on appropriate consumption patterns; and (5) develop, support, and maintain a common evidence base. The EU shows greater interest in limiting demand and harm than in controlling supply.

3.5 **The leading and coordinating role of international organizations**

This chapter cannot overlook what other international organizations around the world are doing in the field of addictions, and how these influence the EU and its member states through reports and guidelines. Two international organizations stand out: the UN and the WHO. The former is relevant not only because of its three international conventions—Single Convention on Narcotic Drugs (1961); Convention on Psychotropic Substances (1971); Convention against Illicit Traffic in Narcotic Drugs and Psychotropic Substances (1988)—but also because of UNGASS and UNODC, an office that reports on the situation, challenges, and evolution of drug trafficking and drug consumption worldwide. The WHO's relevance stems from the Framework Convention on Tobacco Control (FCTC). Despite the EC's efforts, the main tool for tackling tobacco issues at an international level is the FCTC, which has been signed and ratified by the EU and all EU member states except the Czech Republic—the Czech Republic considers voluntary agreements with the tobacco industry sufficient. The FCTC regulates various aspects of tobacco, from its production to its marketing, and measures for reducing supply and demand. Moreover, the

EU has passed directives on labelling and advertising (2001/39/EC and 2003/33/EC) but has drawn up no specific legislative document on tobacco dependence, giving up smoking, education, communication, training, and public awareness (Faid and Gleicher 2011).

Regarding alcohol, WHO's relevance stems from the WHO Expert Committees on Drugs and Alcohol, and on Drug Dependence, the European Alcohol Action Plan, and the 'Global strategy to reduce the harmful use of alcohol'.

Another organization that should be mentioned is the International Narcotics Control Board (INCB), 'an independent and quasi-judicial monitoring body for the implementation of the United Nations international drug control conventions' (INCB 2012).

Finally, the Pompidou Group of the Council of Europe is one of the longest-standing groups—it was established in 1971 at the initiative of the President Pompidou—in the field of drugs and addictions, and noted its work on airport cooperation, focusing on customs and law enforcement, research, information exchange and ad hoc cooperation, drug abuse prevention, and treatment.

3.6 EU achievements: Main common features of the member states' policies

The EU has thus developed a policy based on cooperation whose purpose is to seek a common approach to drug abuse and addictions. We can distinguish two levels of cooperation: the first at the EU level (that is, among member states), and the second between the EU and third countries or regions. While the former began during the 1980s, the latter started at the end of the 1990s and became relevant during the first decade of the twenty-first century through the approval of action plans with third countries and regions.

3.6.1 At EU level

The history of governance of addictions in the EU reveals growing cooperation between member states. Initially, this cooperation was confined to law enforcement, police, and judicial cooperation. Later on, the policy was extended to new health-related domains (among which harm reduction stands out), setting a general EU trend. Even so, member states retain much of their sovereignty on drug and addiction policies.

The main commonalities at the EU level are harm reduction (domestic demand reduction), law enforcement (domestic supply reduction), and internal cooperation. The will to introduce and implement harm reduction policies is a trend that has been boosted by 'an increasing volume of literature criticizing American-style drug policy and research linking a zero-tolerance policy with an increasingly bleak drug problem' (Chatwin 2007: 498). Accordingly, the EU has built a different model for dealing with drugs and addictions from the one found in the USA. Prevention and reduction of drug-related harm is a public-health objective for all EU member states and a major plank in the EU's drugs strategy. Major measures in this field are Opioid Substitution Treatment (OST) and the Needle and Syringe Programme (NSP), which target overdose deaths and the spread of infectious diseases. Substitution treatment and needle and syringe programmes are reported to be available in all EU countries.

The EU has made huge advances toward supply reduction, such as passing the Council Framework Decision 2004/757/JHA, which laid down minimum provisions on the constituent elements of criminal acts and penalties in the field of illicit drug trafficking. However, as seen before in the EU action plans and strategy, supply reduction seems to be a more Europeanized issue than demand reduction, which remains in the hands of member states.

Finally, it is also worth noting that the national drug action plans of many member states developed largely in parallel with those produced by the EU. This is especially relevant when we consider that no fewer than 12 new member states have joined the EU since 2004, many of them from central and eastern Europe. However, through a policy diffusion path and thanks to the EU's 'soft power'—'the ability to get what you want through attraction rather than coer-cion or payments' Nye (2004: 3)—central and eastern EU states have accepted and introduced an EU drugs policy approach into their national policies. Even so, it should be noted that the conditions for membership included adoption of the EU drugs strategy and action plans, introduction of harm reduction as a facet of their national drugs policy, and signing the three UN conventions.

3.6.2 Cooperation between the EU and other countries or regions

Regarding EU external cooperation, the EU drug strategy (2005–2012) under-lines the importance of cooperation with countries on the EU's eastern border, the Balkan states, Afghanistan, and its neighbours. These overarching aims were translated into specific objectives for the EU Drugs Action Plan (2005–2008) and endorsed in 2005, under the headings coordination, supply reduc-tion, and international cooperation.

At the international level, the EU's objective is to speak with one voice in negotiations. The effectiveness of the EU, the world's major donor in the quest for sustainable solutions to the global drug problem, would benefit greatly from better coordination of national and community policies. Moreover, the EU's integrated and balanced approach to drugs is increasingly serving as a model for other countries worldwide (Council of the EU 2008).

3.7 **Conclusion: The EU process. Seeking convergence**

This chapter has focused on the way in which the EU established and institutionalized its policy on drugs and addictions. In the 1980s the EU began to deal with drug issues as the heroin boom and HIV/AIDS started to take their toll. On the one hand, the EU fostered cooperation between member states and standardized its policy on drugs and addictions as far as possible. On the other, it played an important role on the international stage, establishing cooperation agreements with third countries and fostering a model of the governance of addictions.

The Schengen Agreement (1985) also had a big impact, removing frontier controls at a stroke. This was one of the main reasons why the EU started to encourage cooperation between member states, ensuring the dominance of supply-side measures and the law enforcement oriented approach over health-related and harm-reduction policies. The EU expanded its powers throughout the 1990s with the inclusion of drugs in the Maastricht Treaty (1993). It also established a centre for research and monitoring (first CELAD and then EMCDDA). There was a shift away from law enforcement and towards more comprehensive, health-oriented measures. It seemed to be supported by the fact that the Directorate-General for Health and Consumers (DG SANCO) was becoming more involved in the drug field, which had previously been dominated by the Directorate-General for Justice (DG Justice).

The EU approved its first strategies in the twenty-first century (2000–2004 and 2005–2012), presenting a much more comprehensive approach, linking well-being to drugs and addictions, dealing with drug issues as a cross-cutting problem that needed to be tackled from various angles, approving a strategy for alcohol that built on civil society engagement in its formulation, and implementing effective policies. Harm-reducing policies became part of a new trend towards more health-oriented strategies and action plans.

Despite the lack of EU regulation on penalties for possessing, consuming, and trafficking drugs, EU policies in this field have tended to converge over the last three decades (Council of the EU 2004b). Notwithstanding progress in this field, we cannot talk about a formal EU policy on addictions since there is no legal basis for policy-making in this area. Furthermore, the 'search to identify a coherent regional model is also made harder because within all EU member states, as elsewhere, the illicit drugs issue cuts across a spectrum of controversial topics ranging from basic rights and freedoms through public health policies, to criminal justice responses' (Bewley-Taylor 2012: 80). This makes it difficult to reach consensus within a single nation, let alone within the EU. Instead, the EU plays a complementary, supporting role. It is expected to 'add value' to national strategies and, in the medium to long term could manage to standardize national policies and then establish a single EU model for governing addictions. Even so, the new EU drug strategy (2013–2020) reiterates that drug policy is largely a matter for EU member states.

Finally, the influence of international organizations is key to understanding the EU approach's evolution on addictions, particularly the United Nations and the World Health Organization. This is evidenced by the EU and WHO collaborative agreement on monitoring systems, especially tobacco and alcohol.

Note

1 Andalucian Federation; Association Française pour la Réduction des Risques; Association Nationale de Prévention en Alcoologie et Addictologie; Celebrate Recovery (NGO for re-socialization of former addicts); Citywide Drugs Crisis Campaign; De Hoop Foundation; Dianova International; Diogenis; Eurasian Harm Reduction Network; Europe Against Drugs; European AIDS Treatment Group; European Association of Professionals Working in the Drug Field; European Society for Prevention Research; European Treatment Centres for Drug Addiction; European Cities Against Drugs; European Institute of Studies of Prevention; Foundation for a Drug-Free Europe; Fédération Addiction; Fondation Européenne des Services d'Aide Téléphonique Drogue; Forum Européen pour la Sécurité Urbaine; Foundation Regenboog Group; Healthy Options Project Skopje; Hungarian Civil Liberties Union; Institute for Research and Development; International Centre for Antidrugs and Human Rights; International Drug Policy Consortium; International Harm Reduction Association; International Network of People who Use Drugs; Kallódó Ifjúságot Mentő Misszió; Merchant Quay's Ireland; Mentor Foundation; PARSEC Consortium; Placet Agency for Development; San Patrignano Community; Scottish Drug Forum; Spanish Scientific Society for Research on Alcohol; Alcoholism, and other Drug Addictions; Unión de Asociaciones y Entidades de Atención al Drogodependiente; Welfare and Development Association; Women's Organizations Committee on Alcohol and Drug Issues; World Federation Against Drugs.

Chapter 4

Model 1: Trendsetters in illicit substances (Belgium, Czech Republic, Germany, Italy, Luxembourg, the Netherlands, Portugal, Spain)

4.1 Introduction to Model 1

As a result of data gathering, the development of a model to analyse the governance of addictions in Europe (see Fig. 2.3), the elaboration of an in-depth analysis for each of the twenty-eight countries, and the cluster analysis, four models for the governance of addictions in Europe are shown. Chapters 4–7 analyse the characteristics of each of the models and the countries inside the groups.

4.2 Description of the model: Approaches to the governance of addictions

The majority of the countries in model 1 are founding members of the EU. Only Spain and Portugal (1986) and the Czech Republic (2004) became members later. This group of countries has a leading role in Europe not only for having most of the internationally recognized best practices but also for their proactive efforts when dealing with illicit substances and for the introduction of innovative policies (see Box 4.1). All these countries have developed a wide range of policies for prevention, treatment, and harm reduction. This group mainly embraces two of the three trends mentioned in the introduction: decriminalization, and harm reduction. Apart from developing a wide range of policies for prevention and treatment, these countries also follow a health-oriented approach by decriminalizing the possession of illicit substances (mostly cannabis)—small quantities for personal use are regarded as misdemeanours and not a criminal offence (Reuter and Trautmann 2009).

Although none of these countries explicitly uses the term 'well-being' in their national strategies, this model's well-being and relational management approach is explained by their policies towards illicit substances (prevention,

Box 4.1: Key elements of the trendsetters in illicit substances model

- The model is mainly characterized by its strategy towards illicit substances.
- Countries in this model combine a well-being and relational management strategy with a comprehensive structure.
- They share a long trajectory of drugs and addiction legislation.
- They give much importance to harm-reduction policies.
- They have passed laws to decriminalize use and possession of illicit substances.
- They have introduced evidence-based policies to deal with illicit substances, shifting from a repressive to a more liberal approach.
- They are low-rankers in alcohol and tobacco scales: they do not fully include measures related to production, distribution, age limits, taxes, advertising, and marketing.
- Their addictions policy is coordinated between most governmental ministries in the government.
- They decentralize policy-making and implementation to multi-level governance structures (regional and/or local governments).

treatment, harm reduction, social assistance, and reintegration programmes), drug trade related, and drug production related policies. In these countries the focus is mainly on illicit substances. Because of their geopolitical location (on trafficking routes), consumption of illicit substances is high, impacting on public health, which is the main concern of the addictions policies in these countries (see Figs 4.1 and 4.2).

These countries tend to decriminalize possession and heavily implement harm-reduction policies. None of them has supply reduction as a top priority in their aims. This model includes four out of five European countries with injection rooms—countries with injection rooms are Germany, Luxembourg, the Netherlands, Norway, and Spain—a harm-reduction policy that is still poorly implemented because it is a controversial measure.

The countries in this model tend to have loose policies towards the production, distribution, and commercialization of licit substances. They avoid high taxes on alcohol and tobacco, and have not implemented restrictive policies on

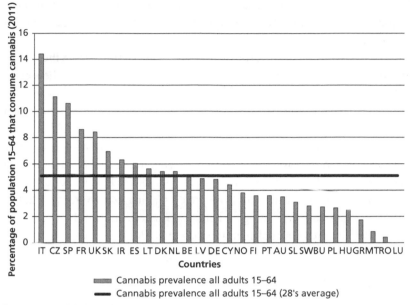

Fig. 4.1 Cannabis prevalence in Europe

Source: data from European Monitoring Centre for Drugs and Drug Addiction (EMCDDA), *Statistical Bulletin—2011*, Copyright © EMCDDA, 1995–2012, available from http://www.emcdda.europa.eu/stats11.

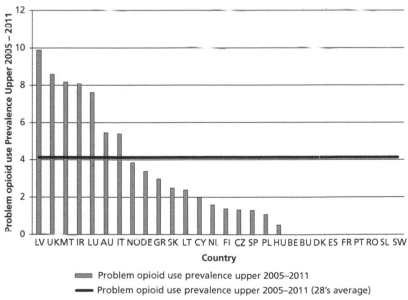

Fig. 4.2 Heroin prevalence in Europe

Source: data from European Monitoring Centre for Drugs and Drug Addiction (EMCDDA), *Statistical Bulletin website*, available from http://www.emcdda.europa.eu/stats13, Copyright © EMCDDA, 1995–2012.

the sponsorship, advertising, and marketing of these products. This is shown by the tobacco and alcohol scales in these countries (see Figs 5.1 and 5.2 in the next chapter).

Countries in this model involve the majority of their ministries in the governance of addictions, because they consider drugs and addictions to be a cross-cutting issue that has to be tackled from different perspectives. They also create an ad hoc body in charge of coordinating the decision-making and implementation process and facilitating exchanges between the many public parties involved throughout the process. This ad hoc body is a platform to coordinate multi-level governance with regions and local governments implementing policies as a way to align activity. The only exceptions are Portugal and Luxembourg, which do not use decentralized policy-making. Finally, these countries have long experience regulating addictive substances and can be regarded as proactive policy-makers implementing top-rated EMCDDA best practices.

4.3 **Germany**

Germany has been traditionally regarded as the growth locomotive of Europe. Moreover, the influence of its policies across the continent has grown since the start of the economic crisis. The German National Strategy on Drug and Addiction Policy adopted in 2012 focuses its attention on 'the avoidance and reduction of the consumption of addictive substances, whether legal or illicit' (Drug Commissioner of the Federal Government 2012: 3). This comprehensive approach is shown in the different areas of action: alcohol, tobacco, prescription drug addiction and prescription drug abuse, pathological gambling, online/media addiction, and illicit drugs. Hence, the strategy not only avoids the division between legal and illicit substances but also includes behavioural addictions such as gambling and media.

Germany embraces most of the characteristics that represent this model (see Annex 15): it has a public-health perspective, decriminalizes drug possession, implements many harm-reduction policies, and still ranks low in scales for legal substances. Furthermore, it has lengthy experience of legislating illicit substances, and devolves policy-making and implementation to decentralized structures. As an exception in this model, the establishment of penalties is not defined according to the classification of substances. Germany, jointly with Portugal, is one of the few countries that involve private sector organizations in the decision-making process, and the single country in the model that embraces the concept of 'addiction' in its national strategy.

Germany passed its first legislation on addictive substances, the German Opium law, known as the *Opiumgesetz*, in 1929 (Lewy 2008). More significant, however, was the 1981 Narcotics Act, aimed at reducing the demand for narcotics and the harm related to addictive substances. The act promoted a public-health perspective linked to prevention, harm reduction, and decriminalization policies, combined with complex but necessary organizational structures and the involvement of different levels of governments, as well as businesses and non-profit stakeholders.

The 2012 national strategy was passed two years after of the Federal Drug Commissioner asked for a federal anti-drug strategy that would standardize German policy on drugs and addictions. The Federal Drug Commissioner is responsible for the addiction policy of the Ministry of Health. The Commission coordinates drug and addiction policies at federal level. The strategy has four main domains of action: prevention; assessment and treatment and help to overcome addiction; harm-reduction measures; and repression. The main priority of the German drug strategy is prevention, and, more specifically, to 'help individuals to avoid and reduce the consumption of legal (alcohol, tobacco and psychotropic pharmaceuticals) and illicit addictive substances' (Germany—EMCDDA Country Overview 2011).

In line with this strategic approach, the Ministry of Health is responsible for addiction policies and the decriminalization of drug possession. In fact, according to German law, non-authorized possession of drugs is a penal crime; however, there are exceptions within German legislation in order to avoid prosecution. These exceptions are linked to the kind and quantity of the substance, the background of the accused, and the degree of public interest in pursuing prosecution. Therefore, in practical terms, Germany decriminalizes possession of illicit substances. Furthermore, Germany includes the establishment of injection rooms among its harm-reduction policy measures.

One of the main issues when analysing Germany is harmonization and coordination across the country's sixteen federal states (*Länder*). The implementation performed by *Länder* and municipalities may have different focuses, under the umbrella of the federal government. In practice, healthcare and social work are governed by the principle of subsidiarity. There are few cases in which the federal government itself provides treatment and services to addicts (counselling facilities run by public-health officers or psychiatric clinics). While the federal government has legislative authority over penal law and laws governing narcotic drugs, penal execution, and social welfare, the *Länder* have the power to execute and implement them. Moreover, the *Länder* also have decision-making powers to legislate on the prevention of illicit substances, especially in areas such as education, health, and schools. Some *Länder* are currently working on shifting some competences (including counselling, care, and general prevention activities) to the municipalities, in order to improve integration between youth welfare and addiction support systems.

Box 4.2: Prevention in Germany: best practices

'Quit the Shit'

'Quit the Shit' was piloted by the Federal Centre for Health Education in 2004 and has since become a highly recognized practice. It is an online withdrawal programme (<http://www.drugcom.de>) aimed at helping young people reduce or quit their cannabis consumption.

Kasse200

It is the largest national programme of education courses for the promotion of health and the prevention of violence and addiction among children aged 6–11. It is one of the oldest programmes (it began in 1991) and its main objective is to promote children's health and skills.

Source: data from European Monitoring Centre for Drugs and Drug Addiction (EMCDDA), *Best Practice Portal*, available from http://www.emcdda.europa.eu/best-practice, Copyright © EMCDDA, 1995–2012

Non-profit organizations play an important role throughout the decision-making and implementation process at national and federal level. Implementation is performed, on the one hand, by social health insurance accredited doctors (general practitioners), tasked to guarantee outpatient medical care, and, on the other hand by charitable organizations providing socio-therapeutic policies for drug users through public funding (either from the German government, the *Länder*, or the municipality).

Prevention is jointly executed and implemented by federal agencies, *Länder*, and the local community. Although the *Länder* share joint responsibility for executing prevention activities with the community, schools are still the most important target institutions for universal prevention, which focuses on alcohol, tobacco, and cannabis. Innovative selective prevention programmes are constantly being developed (see Box 4.2). Further examples are internet-based counselling, phone assessment, and programmes aimed at minority groups. Germany has also indicated prevention programmes mainly focused on children and teenagers with behavioural disorders, and children living in families affected by addiction (Germany—EMCDDA Country Overview 2011).

4.4 Belgium

The first Belgian law on drugs dates back to 1921, one of the oldest of the twenty-eight countries (see Annex 7). Since the approval of the 'drug policy note' of

2011, Belgium tackles legal and illicit substances together with one broad goal: prevent and limit risks for drug users, their environment, and for society as a whole. The policy note establishes the following objectives:

1 To prevent and reduce drug use as well as to decrease the number of new drug users, i.e. prevention of drug consumption.

2 To protect the community and its members, especially those who deal directly or indirectly with the consequences of the drug and addictions phenomenon, i.e. harm reduction, assistance, and reintegration policies.

3 To enforce laws against drug consumption and trafficking. Here it is worth noting that Belgium considers the judicial approach, and imprisonment in particular, as the last option when dealing with problematic use of drugs, i.e. repression as a last resource.

In order to accomplish these objectives and implement a sound policy across the country, the policy note outlines five principles:

1 A comprehensive and integrated approach.

2 Research, epidemiology, and scientific assessment.

3 Prevention of problematic users.

4 Treatment, harm reduction, and reintegration of problematic users.

5 Repression of drug traffickers and producers.

Interestingly, in 2003 Belgium approved a new status for cannabis, the consumption of which is no longer prosecuted unless considered problematic or to be affecting public order. Through a royal decree (2003) Belgium established a legal distinction between possession of cannabis for personal use and any other type of drug-related offence.

The country puts great emphasis on research, epidemiology, and scientific assessment; very few countries put this as the second aim in the national strategy. Like its counterparts in this model, Belgium has soft regulation on tobacco and alcohol.

Belgians still consume primarily beer, although since the 1990s there has been a rise in wine consumption, and alcohol consumption is below the EU average. Tobacco consumption, on the other hand, has increased and is currently above the average for the twenty-eight countries. More specifically, the percentage of smokers in Belgium rose from 26 per cent in 2006 to 30 per cent in 2010, the highest increase within the EU. Finally, it is noteworthy that Belgium, like most of its counterparts in this model, has best practices of the highest attainable standard according to EMCDDA (see Box 4.3).

Since 2009, the Belgian government has had a General Drugs Policy Cell, an inter-ministerial body mandated to coordinate an integrated drug policy in

> ## Box 4.3: The good behaviour game: best practice in Belgium
>
> This measure aims to promote awareness and prevention at an early age (elementary schools). It is done through a classroom-based game that encourages students to manage their own and the team's behaviour. Positive and desirable behaviours are rewarded, undesirable and negative ones are ignored. Implemented from 2006 to 2008, the study's main objective was to 'to investigate the role of the teacher's behaviour management in the development of disruptive behaviour in early elementary school, using a design with a universal classroom preventive intervention' (EMCDDA 2011c).
>
> Source: data from European Monitoring Centre for Drugs and Drug Addiction (EMCDDA), *Best Practice Portal*, available from http://www.emcdda.europa.eu/best-practice, Copyright © EMCDDA, 1995–2012.

Belgium and to support and advise the government. It is composed of seventeen representatives from the federal government and eighteen from regional governments. This ad hoc coordinating body is supported by a research and scientific information cell, which is intended to boost evidence-based policies (Deprez et al. 2011).

The organization, execution, and oversight of preventative activities are in the hands of the regional governments. The implementation of policies and measures diverges, depending on the linguistic community (French, Flemish, and German). The French community tends to turn to associations and specialized services that provide training in schools. The Flemish community, however, prefers a programme-based intervention. Indicated prevention—the focus of which is on individual people, and therefore less emphasis is placed on assessing or addressing environmental influences, such as community values—is increasingly available, especially for the children of addicts in the French community. In the German community neither specialized treatment centres for drug users nor needle exchange programmes are implemented.

4.5 The Czech Republic

The Czech Republic became a member of the EU jointly with most central and eastern European countries (CEECs) in 2004. Once it became a candidate member state of the EU, the Czech Republic started embracing the *acquis communautaire*, harmonizing national legislation at all levels, and including legislation related to drugs to the EU guidelines (see Annex 10). Like its CEEC counter-parts, the Czech Republic did not undertake relevant public policy actions relat-ed to drugs and addictions until the 1990s (EMCDDA 2003), although its first law relating to drugs and addiction dates back to 1962. In that year, just after the approval of the first UN Convention, the Czech authorities passed a Criminal Code and the Criminal Procedure Code aimed at dealing with drug-related offences. But it was not until 1993—the same year the Czech Republic became an independent state through the dissolution of Czechoslovakia—that this country passed its first national strategy. Hence, the Czech Republic's history in drugs could be compared to many western EU countries, whose first laws were approved in the middle of the twentieth century and their first strategies passed at the beginning of the 1990s. The Czech Republic was the first CEEC to accept harm-reduction policies in 1999, when it introduced the concept into the national strategy. Since then, the Czech Republic has deepened its policy on harm reduction.

Although the Czech Republic still embraces some safety and disease approach characteristics—for example, the Ministry of Health is not responsible for tack-ling addictions—it is moving towards a well-being and relational management strategy. And although it is the country with highest prevalence of cannabis consumption (more than double the average prevalence of the twenty-eight countries), it has opted for prosecuting supply. An example of this tendency is that cannabis use has been legal since the 1990s and more recently (2009) can-nabis possession has been decriminalized, sharpening the security focus on manufacturers, importers, and major drug dealers instead of consumers (Global Post 2010). The Czech Republic is thus applying a particular approach, by which countries not only decriminalize use and possession, but also focus on produc-ers and traffickers. The Czech Republic is one of the most liberal countries in the field of decriminalization because it not only determines penalties depend-ing on the substance, but also allows the possession of up to 15g of cannabis and 1.5g of heroin. It is worth noting that the Czech Republic and Hungary are among the few CEECs that have implemented scientific evaluation or impact analysis of their legal changes.

An outstanding characteristic of the Czech Republic's latest national strategy is its long temporal scope, which may help to overcome permanent changes linked to elections and new governments. It was approved in 2010 and it is intended to run until 2018. The aims of this strategy are to:

1 Reduce the level of experimental and occasional drug use, particularly among young people.

2 Reduce the level of problematic and intensive drug use.

3 Reduce potential drug-related risks to individuals and society.

4 Reduce drug availability, particularly to young people.

These objectives are classified in four specific areas: primary prevention, treatment and social reintegration, harm reduction, and reduction of the drug supply. Like the previous national strategy (2005–2009), the new strategy has three main pillars: reducing demand (including prevention and treatment), supply, and harm.

The Czech Republic reports the highest level of alcohol consumption among the EU countries (WHO 2005a), and the largest percentage of smokers in this model, surpassing the average for the twenty-eight countries. Notwithstanding, the Czech Republic implements a strict zero-tolerance drinking and driving policy (BAC = 0.0) and driving under the influence of alcohol can be a criminal offence. However, alcohol taxes are below the EU average, there is no need for a licence to produce beer, wine, or spirits, and licences for selling alcoholic products on-premise or off-premise are not required.

The government's Council for Drug Policy Coordination is responsible for the overall implementation of the national drug strategy and is in charge of initiating, counselling, and coordinating drug issues at government level. Presided over by the prime minister, it is formed by representatives from all the ministries involved in the governance of addictions as well three civil society representatives, the Czech Medical Association, the Association for Addictive Diseases, the Association of NGOs dealing with drug prevention and treatment, and the Association of the Regions (Mravčík et al. 2010).

There is significant multi-level governance in the policy-making and implementation process regarding addictions. The Czech Republic has a network of fourteen regional coordinators focused on implementing the national strategy at regional and local level. The regional authorities make policy, and the local authorities implement prevention, harm-reduction, and treatment policies. The involvement of private and non-profit stakeholders is well established. These organizations are involved in decision-making bodies, such as Government Council for Drug Policy Coordination, and in the implementation process. In this respect, while prevention is mainly developed through state schools, non-profit and public organizations deliver most of the treatment policies. The Secretariat of the Council of the Government for Drug Policy Coordination organizes the distribution of subsidies to service providers in the sphere of treatment of drug addiction and reintegration.

4.6 Italy

Until 2006 Italy could have been said to have a de facto decriminalization policy. However, since 2006 Italian justice and law enforcement have become stricter and possession of any substance (including cannabis) can be considered and punished as drug trafficking. This shift could have been due to the new government of Prime Minister Romano Prodi after the 2006 elections and the high prevalence of cannabis and heroin, which is significantly above the average for the twenty-eight countries. Italian penalties for the possession and trafficking of opiates or addictive barbiturates are stricter than the EU recommendations (Council of the EU 2004b). In addition, despite the focus on illicit substances, the national strategy also introduced many preventative actions for legal substances.

The Italian policy focus is on prevention followed by treatment and harm reduction; however, drug and addiction polices do not come under the Ministry of Health (see Annex 19). Instead, a presidential department is mandated to develop and coordinate this policy. Italy has created an ad hoc National Committee of Anti-Drug Policy, composed of ministries and reporting to the Presidential Sub-secretary of the Ministers' Council. The committee is in charge of setting national planning, but also coordinates the work of the ministries and regions involved in the policy-planning and implementation process. This is done through the Committee of State Regions and the Committee of Municipal Regions. At regional level, drug and addictions policies are also coordinated through the Regional Office of Drugs and Drug Addiction, which reports to the Department of Social Policy and Health.

The National Committee excludes alcohol and takes a holistic approach. However, it has an action plan for alcohol that was approved by the Ministry of Health in 2007. Taking into account policy and control scales, we note that Italy still rates way below the EU average in alcohol policy scales, although consumption levels are also below the average for the twenty-eight countries. Italy is the only Mediterranean country that implements zero tolerance policies for professional and novice drivers. As with alcohol, tobacco-control scales rate below the average, but the percentage of smokers and cigarettes consumed per day are also below the average. In this respect, lower ratings in control scales do not necessarily imply that a country will have high levels of consumption.

In Italy, harm-reduction measures are focused on preventing the use and abuse of substances, but not on reducing the harm caused by these substances once consumed. Prevention, the main focus of the Italian policy, is mainly provided by the regions, which develop their own plans; nonetheless, half of the funding of universal and selective prevention comes from the national government. In prevention, the most important budgets go to education and support for families, early diagnosis, and behavioural neuroscience (see Box 4.4). Treatment is also decentralized, and it is provided by regions and local institutions, although the national government funds these activities. Families are highly

---

Box 4.4: Prevention in Italy: best practice

Unplugged

From 2004 to 2007 Italy implemented a school-based programme targeted at 12–14-year-olds. The main objective was to reduce the take-up, use, and abuse of tobacco, alcohol, and other illicit substances, stopping the transition from consumption to addiction.

Source: data from European Monitoring Centre for Drugs and Drug Addiction (EMCDDA), *Best Practice Portal*, available from http://www.emcdda.europa.eu/best-practice, Copyright © EMCDDA, 1995–2012.

---

involved in prevention tasks in various ways, such as mutual assistance, family meetings, and family training.

4.7 Luxembourg

Luxembourg is the smallest country within this model. However, it has the highest GDP per capita of the twenty-eight countries in the sample and reports the highest rate in OECD material living conditions (see Annex 22). The country takes a holistic perspective on addictions, which is not substance specific. The current national strategy has two pillars—reduction of supply and demand—with four axes: reduction of risk damage and nuisance; research and information; international relations; and coordination mechanisms. Notwithstanding, the main focus is on primary prevention, socio-professional reinsertion measures, diversification, and access to therapeutic offers and quality management. There is ministerial division of responsibilities: while the Ministry of Health is responsible for demand reduction, risk reduction, and research, the Ministry of Justice and the Ministry of Foreign Affairs are in charge of supply reduction and international cooperation respectively.

Luxembourg follows a public-health approach, decriminalizing cannabis use, and implementing harm-reduction policies (included needle exchange in prisons), but without extensive regulation for legal substances. More specifically, it ranks among the lowest on the alcohol policy scales and is among the three countries with the lowest tobacco control scale (only surpassed by Austria and Greece). Luxembourg has an ad hoc coordinator body, the Inter-ministerial Commission on Drugs (ICDL), which is the top decision-level entity with respect to coordination and orientation of actions. The coordinator and some representatives of this body are appointed by the Ministry of Health, while the rest of the commission is composed of senior delegates from the main governmental departments.

This centralized structure does not impede the active involvement of non-profit organizations. More specifically, there are state-accredited non-governmental organizations that provide treatment throughout the country. The active involvement of non-profit organizations in the implementation process is controlled by coordination platforms composed of the non-profit organizations and a representative from the ministry. Furthermore, the ICDL's coordinator meets periodically with non-profit organizations in order to follow up the implementation of policies, share information, and devise responses to emergent situations (Origer 2009).

Due to its low tobacco price, Luxembourg has been accused of 'exporting cancer', and the Association of European Leagues against Cancer ranks this country twenty-ninth out of thirty-one states. In this respect, Luxembourg is a clear example of a country that on the one hand has innovative policies towards decriminalization and harm reduction (it is one of the few EU countries with injection rooms), but very soft controls and regulatory measures on legal substances (tobacco and alcohol). Luxembourg has hardly any alcohol measures in force, and is thus one of the most alcohol liberal countries in the EU.

4.8 **The Netherlands**

Leaving the exceptional case of Luxembourg aside, the Netherlands has the highest GDP per capita and highest rates in euros/inhabitant (see Annex 24). It also performs well in OECD indicators (well-being, status, and management indexes), risk poverty, the GINI Index, and the Corruption Perception Index. The Netherlands was first categorized as a Nordic country by Esping-Andersen due to its balanced combination of equity (high expenditure on social protection) and efficiency (low unemployment levels).

The legislation on illicit drugs is based on the country's Opium Law, a by-product of the 1912 International Opium Convention held at The Hague. However this law was radically amended in 1972, distinguishing between hard and soft drugs and introducing a risk scale based on medical, pharmacological, sociological, and psychological data. Illicit classification of substances is split into 'substances presenting unacceptable risks' and 'other substances'. The last drug policy letter published in May 2011, during Prime Minister Mark Rutte's administration, establishes two pillars: public-health protection and the fight against public nuisance and organized crime. Thus the priority for the Netherlands is still prevention, followed by harm reduction, treatment, and social assistance.

The main ministry in charge of dealing with illicit drugs and addictions and tasked with the coordination of drug policy is the Ministry of Health, Welfare, and Sports, followed by the Ministry of Security and Justice and the Ministry of Foreign Affairs. These ministries follow four broad objectives:

1 Prevent drug use; treat and rehabilitate drug users.

2 Reduce harm to users.

3 Diminish public nuisance caused by drug users.

4 Combat the production and trafficking of drugs.

The country determines penalties according to drug classification, decriminalizes possession, has injection rooms, does not prioritize supply reduction measures in its strategy, and has top-rated best practices. However, the Netherlands does not have an ad hoc body coordinating addiction policies, a characteristic that is shared only by Denmark out of the twenty-eight countries in the sample. The Netherlands stands out for being the only country of our sample with top-rated EMCDDA best practices in prevention, treatment, and harm-reduction policies. More specifically, it is the only country with top-rated best practices in the treatment and harm-reduction domain, since the best practices of the rest of the countries are found in prevention (see Box 4.5).

Box 4.5: The Netherlands: top-rated best practices in the treatment and harm-reduction domain

Treatment

'Family motivational intervention' treats cannabis consumers with onset of schizophrenia and aims to reduce cannabis use, increase medication compliance, increase the well-being of parents, reduce the stress the family experiences in relation to schizophrenic disorders and improve communication between parents and children.

Harm reduction

There is only one policy action rated a 3 by the EMCDDA. This is implemented by the Netherlands and known as 'low threshold supportive care for local, treatment-avoiding and inaccessible polydrug users with problematic crack use'. This harm-reduction-oriented policy aims to reduce public-health risk and public nuisance related to crack use.

Source: data from European Monitoring Centre for Drugs and Drug Addiction (EMCDDA), *Best Practice Portal*, available from http://www.emcdda.europa.eu/best-practice, Copyright © EMCDDA, 1995–2012.

As has every country in this model, the Dutch government has decriminalized the possession of drugs, and even its use, especially for consumers of substances such as cannabis. Despite its cannabis policy, and its well-known 'coffee shops', the Netherlands reports levels of cannabis prevalence on average or even below that of the twenty-eight countries. Many countries in this model give a lot of attention to the promotion of evidence-based interventions through the collaboration of different centres. In the Netherlands, these include the Centre for Healthy Living of the National Institute of Public Health and the Trimbos Institute.

The Netherlands has developed national strategies and action plans for illicit drugs and has also established programmes for alcohol and tobacco. Hence, this country does not merge policies on legal and illicit substances, which is why it cannot be regarded as having a comprehensive structure for dealing with addictions. The Netherlands is also characterized by decentralized policy-making and implementation with multi-level governance. For instance, prevention is funded by the Ministry of Health but mainly conducted by municipalities in collaboration with schools and other non-profit organizations. Treatment is also managed by decentralized structures, which co-produce these policies in collaboration with regional non-profit organizations and businesses.

4.9 **Portugal**

Portugal has been a pioneer in introducing decriminalization policies. More specifically, in 2001 it became the first European country officially to abolish all criminal penalties for use and possession of drugs, including cannabis, cocaine, heroin, and methamphetamine. According to Szalavitz (2009), the argument defending this position is that imprisoning addicts is more expensive than treatment and further alienates this population, so it is more beneficial to provide health services instead. This decriminalization policy has been implemented by many other countries around the globe; hence the Portuguese case has been extensively studied by experts in the field.

The notion of drug decriminalization was first introduced in Portugal in 1976 by the Youth Studies Centre (the Centro de Estudos da Juventude focuses on developing prevention and treatment research), which noted that 'the concept of drug use should be revised and replaced when justified, by a set of norms to bring it under an administrative offence framework. The response to drug use would thus move from a criminal penalty model towards clinical treatment and the qualification of the drug user as a patient and not as a criminal' (Trigueiros et al. 2010, cited in Portugal—EMCDDA Portugal Profile 2011: 11). In 1993, in parallel with the first Portuguese law on supply reduction, the Portuguese parliament questioned criminalization and called for a wider policy consensus better to implement the national strategies (Dias 2007). It was not until 1999 that Portugal approved the national strategy that would lay the groundwork for the drugs and addictions policy of this country and many others.

The strategy was the final output of the Commission for the National Strategy to Fight against Drugs, which was established by the Portuguese government in 1998 to deal with problematic heroin consumption and HIV transmission. The report (1999), which remains the foundation of today's drug policy in Portugal, presented 13 strategic options to guide public action in the drugs field:

> (1) reinforce international cooperation; (2) decriminalize (but still prohibit) drug use; (3) focus on primary prevention; (4) assure access to treatment; (5) extend harm reduction interventions; (6) promote social reintegration; (7) develop treatment and harm reduction in prisons; (8) develop treatment as an alternative to prison; (9) increase research and training; (10) develop evaluation methodologies, (11) simplify interdepartmental coordination; (12) reinforce the fight against drug trafficking and money laundering; (13) double public investment in the drugs field.
> (Portugal—EMCDDA Policy Profile 2011: 15–16)

In this sense, the national strategy of 2005–2012 follows the guidelines of this report while introducing a few novelties, such as local planning and management, improving the coordination and integration of service providers, focusing on users' needs, and improving the quality of the service through accreditation mechanisms.

When looking at how decriminalization policies have affected Portuguese levels of consumption we see that cannabis prevalence is below the EU average and reports the lowest level of this model (see Annex 27). This can be seen as a success of the decriminalization policy since Portugal, like Spain, is a European gateway for cocaine and cannabis (CIA 2012). As a result of decriminalizing drug use and drug possession, users stop being afraid of the judicial system and lose their fear of asking for help. Furthermore, police forces become able to focus on relevant high-level dealers trafficking large quantities of drugs (Szalavitz, 2009). Related to this, a report published by Greenwald (2009: 15) found that in 'the five years after personal possession was decriminalized, illicit drug use among teens in Portugal declined and rates of new HIV infections caused by sharing of dirty needles dropped, while the number of people seeking treatment for drug addiction more than doubled'.

The Portuguese policy approach forced a change of ministry in charge of this field. EMCDDA (2011a: 23) identifies that Portugal has 'progressively removed responsibilities from the Ministry of Justice to give them to the Ministry of Health'. This has to ensure that 'any Portuguese citizen faced with a substance abuse problem, including alcohol, tobacco, and medicines should be considered holistically in terms of Ministry responses' (EMCDDA 2011a: 21). Furthermore, in 2006 Portugal established the Institute on Drugs and Drug Addiction (IDT), an ad hoc body mandated to conduct policy coordination as well as planning, managing, monitoring, and evaluating prevention, treatment, and rehabilitation of both drugs and alcohol. It reports to the Ministry of Health and is charged with implementing actions established in the national strategy and action plans.

Portugal also has the National Council for the Fight Against Drugs, Drug Addiction and the Harmful Use of Alcohol, an advisory body chaired by the Minister of Health and composed of five experts appointed by the government representing regional government, the judiciary, the General Prosecutor, and civil society. This body provides advice to the government on national strategies and actions plans and follows reports of their implementation. Despite the fact that decisions on drugs and addictions are taken by the central government, local entities and stakeholders are very important and taken into account in the implementation process, looking for synergy partnerships with local communities in order to address their problems properly. It is notable that the central government has established 163 areas based on drugs and addictions criteria instead of administrative criteria.

As a matter of principle, the Portuguese national strategy includes citizens' engagement and the establishment of partnerships that help to identify the community's needs. Quoting the EMCDDA (Portugal—EMCDDA Country Overview 2011), 'in each specific territory, an intervention may address different problems and bring together different partners, working in different settings, depending on the identified needs'. An example of these partnerships can be seen in treatment services, which are provided by a large network of public, private, and non-profit organizations.

The relevance of local entities can be seen by looking at the Commission for the Dissuasion of Drug Abuse, a local commission that implements decriminalization policies by evaluating drug-related cases and assessing whether there is any suspicion of drug trafficking. Despite decriminalization policies, penalties for illicit drug trafficking linked to criminal organizations may be as much as up to twenty-five years' imprisonment, which outweighs by fifteen years the EU recommendations (Council of the EU 2004b). This means that Portuguese sanctions for trafficking with aggravating circumstances are higher than the EU's recommendations.

The action plan 2009–2012 (Institute on Drugs and Drug Addiction 2009) is oriented to demanding reduction through prevention, deterring addiction, treatment, harm reduction, and social reintegration. The relevance of prevention

Box 4.6: Portugal's best practices in the field of prevention

Searching Family Treasure

With the intention of reducing risk factors and increase protective factors, this programme targets at-risk families with children aged between 6 and 12, and offers skills programmes and individual support.

Grow Up Playing: a prevention programme for primary schools

This school-based programme for children between 6 and 10 promotes protective factors and aims to reduce risk factors through cartoons, games, and activities.

Source: data from European Monitoring Centre for Drugs and Drug Addiction (EMCDDA), *Best Practice Portal*, available from http://www.emcdda.europa.eu/best-practice, Copyright © EMCDDA, 1995–2012.

policies is confirmed by the fact that Portugal has top-rated best practices in prevention (see Box 4.6). Besides, actions on demand reduction outweigh those aimed at reducing supply of substances.

The three main objectives in prevention are:

1 Increase the number of drug prevention programmes based on scientific evidence.

2 Increase the number of selective prevention programmes aimed at vulnerable groups.

3 Improve the selection process, monitoring, and evaluation of prevention programmes.

Despite its holistic approach, the Portuguese National Plan against drugs and drug addictions (2005–2012) still tackles legal and illicit substances separately (Institute on Drugs and Drug Addiction 2005), and ranks low on tobacco and alcohol policy scales. Nonetheless, the advisory body chaired by the Ministry of Health and the IDT is starting to consider both kinds of substance together, placing the focus on addictions instead of substances. On the other hand, in 2006, the IDTs' mandate was extended in order to conduct policy coordination, planning, management, monitoring, and evaluation of prevention, treatment, and rehabilitation of legal and illicit substances.

4.10 **Spain**

Following the trend of Mediterranean countries, Spain reports fewer than five out of ten OECD material living condition indicators (2011) and its GDP per capita is slightly below the EU mean. Spain stands out for having the highest unemployment rates—both for the overall population (21.7 per cent) and among young people (46.4 per cent)—of the twenty-eight countries analysed (see Annex 31).

In Spain, the Ministry of Health is in charge of drug policy, the classification of drugs determines the final penalties, and cannabis possession is decriminalized; it is one of the few countries to have injection rooms. Spain suffered a huge epidemic of HIV/AIDS drug-related deaths in the 1990s that resulted in it becoming one of the most innovative countries in harm-reduction strategies. However, it rates below the mean of the twenty-eight countries on the alcohol policy scale and its score on the tobacco control scale is lower than the mid-point.

Until 2003 Spain dealt with drugs and addiction through the Ministry of the Interior. That year the government shifted its approach towards a public-health strategy and placed the governance of addictions under the responsibility of the Ministry of Health. Much as Italy and Portugal, however, Spain imposes higher penalties than the EU recommendations when large quantities or aggravating circumstances are involved.

We cannot ignore the fact that Spain is the main entry point for cannabis coming from North Africa, especially Morocco, into the EU. This means that the Spanish cannabis market is wide and the price is low. This accounts for why cannabis consumption in Spain is practically twice as much as the EU average. As in Portugal, Spanish legislation for cannabis is less strict than the EU average; consumption is not illicit and possession for personal consumption is considered an administrative offence.

Apart from decriminalization, the National Plan on Drugs identifies prevention as a priority area of action in this country, especially prevention based on education, aimed at young people, and implemented through schools and colleges. Jointly with the Netherlands, Spain is the country with most top-rated best practices in the field of prevention (see Box 4.7). Most prevention measures in Spain are universal, being selective measures on a second term, and indicated prevention is almost residual.

On the other hand, the consumption of legal substances has not been regarded as problematic. Spain is a wine producer country and during the 1960s it was classified as wine drinking country. According to the WHO (2011a), beer consumption has increased and is now higher than wine consumption (45 per cent

Box 4.7: Spanish preventive best practices

Brief intervention in alcohol-related traffic accidents

Targeted at non-alcoholic drinkers, this practice aims to reduce traffic accidents related to alcohol consumption. More specifically, the programme takes 'advantage of the opportunity presented by the traffic accident to influence the drinking behaviour of non-alcoholics, especially in relation to driving, through a brief counselling intervention at the hospital' EMCDDA (2011c).

Emotions, Thoughts, and Feelings for Healthy Development

EmPeCemos aims to prevent behavioural problems and drug abuse among children aged 7–10. Determined as a key predictor of drug abuse, the programme targets this at an early stage. It focuses on family, school, and children's skills and aims to promote social competence and break the 'circle of cumulative impairments of disruptive children' EMCDDA (2011c).

Source: data from European Monitoring Centre for Drugs and Drug Addiction (EMCDDA), *Best Practice Portal*, available from http://www.emcdda.europa.eu/best-practice, Copyright © EMCDDA, 1995–2012.

and 36 per cent respectively of the total alcohol consumption). Nowadays, Spain still consumes less alcohol than the average of the twenty-eight countries. It is aligned with the Mediterranean pattern as defined by Anderson et al. (2012) and characterized by rating below the mean of the twenty-eight on the alcohol policy scale. Tobacco consumption, however, is higher than the average among the twenty-eight; according to Joossens and Raw (2010), tobacco control activities are poorly funded and smoke-free legislation in the workplace is weakly enforced.

Spain has a long history and extensive experience in regulating illicit substances (since 1978), has had an ad hoc coordinator body since 1985 (the National Plan on Drugs), and devolves policy-making and implementation to the regions (*comunidades autónomas*). Like many of the twenty-eight, this institution aims to coordinate and enhance drug and addictions policies carried out by public administrations and social organizations. However, the implementation process is performed by the regions, which also have the capacity to determine policies and measures to govern addictions. In this sense, policy implementation is highly decentralized and regional governments have much

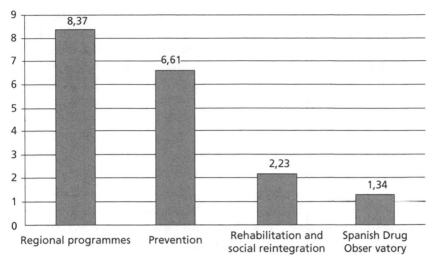

Fig. 4.3 The Spanish national plan on drugs, 2011 budget (€million)

Source: data from Spanish Ministry of Health and Social Affairs, *Spanish Drug Action Plan 2009–2012*, Spanish Government - Ministry of Health and Social Affairs, Spain, Copyright © 2009.

power and control over policies. Most regional governments have the following resources to implement their drug and addictions policy: ambulatory centres for assistance, hospital detoxification units, therapeutic communities, methadone programmes centres, clinical trials with heroin, buprenorphine programmes, and harm-reduction programmes (Spain—EMCDDA Country Overview 2011). The high level of decentralization can also be seen in the budget for the Spanish National Plan on Drugs (see Fig. 4.3), where the largest budgetary item is for the regions, followed by prevention.

4.11 **Conclusion to Model 1 in Europe**

This model groups Continental and Mediterranean welfare states (Esping-Andersen 1990; Ferrera 1996). Notwithstanding this classification, and despite the different contextual levels found in each group of countries, all can be classified as having a well-being and relational management strategy combined with a comprehensive structure.

However, the key domain in this case has been strategy, in which the eight countries rate very similarly and have been classified together in the different methodologies used. In this respect, all these countries have developed well-being-oriented policies and most make the Ministry of Health the responsible institution, giving much weight to harm-reduction policies, decriminalizing possession of illicit substances with few exceptions, proactively developing policies aimed at coping with drug-related problems, embracing a health-oriented rather than a security-oriented approach, and protecting the public and society in general instead of the individual. Thus, almost all these countries have a long history of legislating for illicit substances, and their policy path has been consistent throughout the last three decades. Furthermore, half of these countries have injection rooms and almost all implement top-rated best practices (EMCDDA 2011c), which can be regarded as proactive and innovative policies to deal with the drugs and addictions.

Due to their geopolitical location and the levels of consumption reported, countries within model 1, trendsetters in illicit substances, are characterized by prioritizing policies and measures related to illicit substances, and relegating the regulation of legal substances to a secondary level. This decision is based on the fact that the main problem for most of these countries is illicit substances (cannabis, heroin, cocaine, and synthetic drugs), while problems related to legal substances are less prominent. The only exception in this group is the Czech Republic. Moreover, most of these countries are wine or beer producers, and some, for example, Spain and Italy, are among the top tobacco producers. In this respect, it might be more difficult for them to tighten regulations on legal substances, since their national industries exercise lobby pressures to prevent that.

Chapter 5

Model 2: Regulation of legal substances (Finland, France, Ireland, Norway, Sweden, UK)

5.1 Description of the model: Approaches to the governance of addictions

This cluster contains countries with high rates in non-material as well as economic indicators. In fact, the Nordic countries report the highest scores in five out of eleven variables taken into account by the OECD Better Life Initiative (OECD 2011a). They also report better than the EU average in GDP per capita, personal income, and inequality indicators, as well as in the Corruption Perception Index and sustainable governance indicators (2011). However, we see notorious differences between the Nordic countries on the one hand, and the Anglo-Saxon countries and France on the other, the former having better scores in almost all the variables taken into account. In this sense, it is worth noting that Ireland is the only country within this model with traditional rather than rational values (World Values Survey 2012).

As noted by Anderson et al. (2012), there are two patterns of alcohol consumption within this cluster that distinguishes the Nordic from the Anglo-Saxon countries and France. The level of alcohol consumption in Finland, Norway, and Sweden is below the EU average, while the UK, Ireland, and France report higher levels of alcohol consumption, both recorded and unrecorded, than the EU average (see Fig. 5.1.).

Traditional Nordic patterns of consumption have been characterized by non-daily drinking and irregular heavy and very heavy drinking episodes (mainly of spirits), with the acceptance of public drunkenness (Anderson et al. 2012). On the other hand, in the central-western country model, people tend to prefer beer (wine in France) to spirits, and the levels of acceptance of public drunkenness are not as high as in the Nordic countries, although the UK and Ireland are closer to the Nordic countries than to central-western countries in this respect. Finally, we can also distinguish two models of alcohol production and commercialization: on the one hand, the Nordic model is characterized by an alcohol monopoly in which a government enterprise controls the manufacture and/or

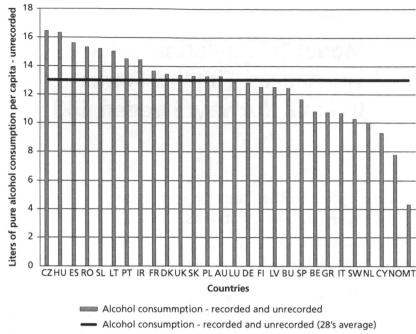

Fig. 5.1 Per capita consumption of pure alcohol per year in Europe

Source: data from World Health Organization (WHO), *Global information system on alcohol and health: levels of consumption,* available at http://apps.who.int/gho/data/node.main, Copyright © WHO 2013 and World Health Organization (WHO), *Levels of Consumption: Recorded adult per capita consumption, from 1961, Total by country,* available at http://apps.who.int/gho/data/node.main.A1025?lang=en?showonly=GISAH, Copyright © WHO 2013.

retail of some alcoholic beverages; on the other hand, the Anglo-Saxons and France have a much more liberalized market.

Levels of consumption of tobacco are quite similar (see Fig. 5.2), although we can still distinguish the same two groups (Nordic and Anglo-Saxon). However, the differentiation between the two groups is not as clear as it is for alcohol consumption. While the Nordic group tends to have lower levels of consumption than the average for the twenty-eight for all substances, the Anglo-Saxons report either similar or slightly higher levels of substance consumption. Ireland stands out for being the only country within the model that has a percentage of smokers above the mean for the twenty-eight.

Cannabis consumption varies depending on the country under study and, interestingly, we can distinguish the same two groups found for alcohol (see Fig. 4.1). Thus, whereas the UK, France, and Ireland report higher levels of cannabis consumption than the average for the twenty-eight, the prevalence of the

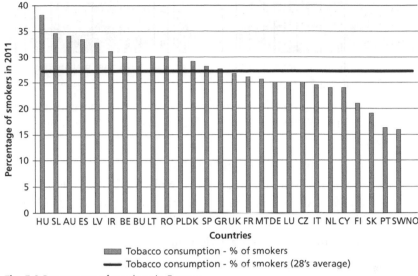

Fig. 5.2 Percentage of smokers in Europe

Source: data from Eurostat website, available at http://appsso.eurostat.ec.europa.eu/nui/
submitViewTableAction.do, Copyright © European Union, 1995–2011.

remaining countries is significantly below the mean (around four percentage
points). This pattern of grouping the Nordic countries on the one hand, the
Anglo-Saxon countries and France on the other is not reproduced when analysing heroin consumption, which varies in each of the countries (see Fig. 4.2). In
this case, we see that the United Kingdom and Finland report the highest levels,
while the rest of the countries have lower levels of prevalence and no reliable
data have been found for Sweden and France.

All the countries in this model have a comprehensive rather than a substance-
based structure (see Box 5.1). Furthermore, this group of countries could be
considered as having a well-being and relational management strategy. In fact,
if they are not fully labelled as that and grouped with the former model, it is
because they place an emphasis on evidence-based regulation of legal substances vs illicit substances, policies of decriminalization, and harm reduction. In
this sense, the main commonality of this model is the significant degree and
number of evidence-based regulatory policies. In fact, out of the twenty-eight
countries, these six are the only ones with high rates of alcohol and tobacco
scales (see Figs 5.3 and 5.4), which embrace an evidence-based regulative
approach aimed at reducing the levels of consumption while pursuing improvement of the quality of life for society as a whole.

Box 5.1: Key elements of the regulation of legal substances model

- Their policies for legal substances are aligned with the 'well-being and relational management' strategy.
- Countries in the model have a comprehensive structure that is combined, at least for legal substances, with a 'well-being and relational management' approach.
- Have a sound trajectory for dealing with drugs.
- Focus on legal substances: the countries implement evidence-based regulations aimed at reducing the levels of alcohol and tobacco consumption. They rank above the mean in both alcohol and tobacco scales.
- Their aim is to enhance societal well-being.
- Their means is by preventing heavy use over time and improving the overall well-being of the population.
- None of the six countries decriminalizes illicit substances.
- Implementation is decentralized; countries in this model also involve non-profit organizations in the decision-making.

Only two countries decriminalize possession of illicit substances (Finland and Ireland) and Norway is the only country to have injection rooms. Furthermore, the UK and Ireland are the only countries that determine penalties according to the legal classification of illicit substances, and are among the few countries that have supply reduction as one of the top priorities in their national strategy.

All this can explain why these countries rate lower than those in model 1 on strategy—they do not embrace the policies most aligned with a well-being and relational management approach. None of these countries identifies public health as a priority in the national strategy. In summary, they fall into the same cluster specifically because of the strategy items. In this respect, as in the first model, we can affirm that strategy characteristics are determinant and the most relevant ones to establish the final cluster. Thus, structure follows strategy.

It is worth noting that most of the countries within this model are more focused on providing treatment and prevention than on implementing harm-reduction policies. This policy measure is still underdeveloped, compared to countries in model 1. These countries approach the regulation of illicit substances by establishing strict laws for drug trade and drug production,

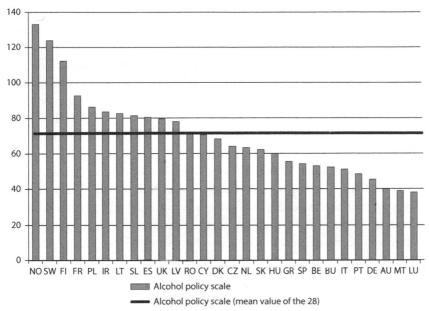

Fig. 5.3 Alcohol policy scale in Europe

Source: data from Karlsson, T. et al., Does alcohol policy make any difference? Scales and consumption, in P. Anderson et al. (eds), *Alcohol Policy in Europe: Evidence from AMPHORA,* The AMPHORA project, Copyright © 2012, available from www.amphoraproject.net/view.php?id_cont=45.

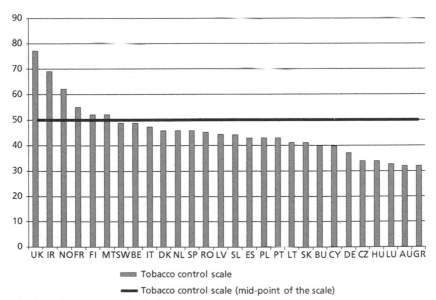

Fig. 5.4 Tobacco-control scale in Europe

Source: data from Joossens, L. and Raw, M., *The Tobacco Control Scale 2010 in Europe,* Association of the European Cancer Leagues, Belgium, Copyright © 2010 Association of European Cancer Leagues.

and imposing higher penalties than the EU recommendation, with the exception of France and Finland, which follow the Council recommendations and are not as restrictive as their counterparts.

Therefore these countries have undertaken more control through evidence-based regulatory policies. This approach is clear in the case of legal substances, which are governed by regulations limiting the retail, distribution, and consumption of tobacco and alcohol. However, their approach towards illicit substances prevents us from classifying this group of countries as having a well-being and relational management strategy.

All the six countries in model 2 have an ad hoc body, decentralize policy implementation, and focus on addictions in general instead of specific substances in their national documents. Moreover, we find that most of these countries tackle legal and illicit substances together, involve non-profit organizations in the decision-making process, and have long experience of legislating drug-related issues.

5.2 **Sweden**

Sweden performs very well in most OECD Better Life Initiative variables and has the highest EU score in governance, health, and environment (see Annex 32). Moreover, it rates above the mean for the twenty-eight in GDP per capita and income, and its unemployment and inequality indicators are below the average. Interestingly, this country obtains the highest rate in status and management indexes (Sustainable Governance Indicators 2011). Sweden has a long tradition of implementing policies on addictions and is regarded by many experts in the field as a model in itself. In fact, Sweden has traditionally had the ambition to export its approach to other EU countries, and has been legitimized by its low levels of addictive substance consumption. The UNODC (2007) states that the 'clear association between a restrictive drug policy and low-levels of drug use is striking'.

As stated in the 2011–2015 strategy ('A cohesive strategy for alcohol, narcotic drugs, doping and tobacco policy'), Sweden pursues a society:

> free from illicit drugs and doping, with reduced alcohol-related medical and social harm, and reduced tobacco use. The objective entails: zero tolerance towards illicit drugs and doping, measures aimed at reducing all tobacco use and deterring minors from starting to use tobacco, prevention of all harmful consumption of alcohol, e.g. by reducing consumption and harmful drinking habits.
> (Swedish Ministry of Health and Social Affairs 2011: 6)

Apart from this broad objective, the strategy has seven long-term goals:

1 Curtailing the supply of illicit drugs, doping substances, alcohol, and tobacco.

2 Protecting children from the harmful effects of alcohol, narcotic drugs, doping, and tobacco.

3 Gradually reducing the number of children and young people who initiate the use of tobacco, narcotic drugs or doping substances, or begin drinking alcohol early.

4 Gradually reducing the number of people who become involved in harmful use, abuse, or dependence on alcohol, illicit drugs, doping substances, or tobacco.

5 Improving access by people with abuse or addiction problems to good quality care and support.

6 Reducing the number of people who die or suffer injuries or damage to their health as a result of their own or others' use of alcohol, narcotic drugs, doping substances, or tobacco.

7 Promoting a public-health based, restrictive approach to alcohol, narcotic drugs, doping, and tobacco in the EU and internationally (Swedish Ministry of Health and Social Affairs 2011: 4).

An outstanding feature of this strategy, also seen in France, Ireland, and Norway, is the aim of tackling legal and illicit substances through a single and cohesive approach. Thus, as stated in the strategy (Swedish Ministry of Health and Social Affairs 2011: 3), 'by adopting a cohesive, integrated approach, the government aims to clarify its intention to deal with the problems that the use and abuse of alcohol, narcotic drugs, doping substances, and tobacco pose as a whole, both to the individual and to society at large'. This quotation presents the country's comprehensive goal to go beyond the individual in order to protect society at large.

Like all the countries in the regulation of legal substances model, the Ministry of Health (and Social Affairs, in Sweden) is responsible for deciding policies on drugs and addictions. There are five pillars to the strategy: prevention, treatment, rehabilitation, protection of children and teens, and supply reduction. It does not give the same attention to harm reduction as a long-term objective. Harm-reduction policies deal with alcohol, tobacco, narcotics, doping, and heroin. It was not until 2006 that the Swedish government passed a law allowing the counties to introduce needle exchange programmes. However, these programmes cannot be implemented without the authorization of the Swedish National Board of Health and Welfare.

Notwithstanding, Sweden has been characterized as having a restrictive policy on addictions. It was only in the first decade of this century that Sweden liberalized its integral alcohol monopoly; nowadays it only keeps an alcohol monopoly in retail off-licences through the *Systembolaget* (System Company), the national authority mandated to control off-licence sales. The *Systembolaget* is a government-owned retail chain and the outlet allowed to sell alcoholic beverages containing 3.5 per cent of alcohol or more. Apart from the *Systembolaget*, alcohol in Sweden is highly regulated through licences, off-licence sales, and police and municipal supervision of sales in licensed premises. Moreover, the legal age to buy alcohol on licensed premises is 18, and 20 for off-licences. The *Konsumentverket* agency, from the Ministry of Agriculture, Food, and Consumer Affairs, controls the marketing and sponsoring of alcoholic beverages shown on television, on the radio, in the cinema, in printed media, on advertising hoardings, in sport stadiums, and on sportswear; it also establishes place, day, and time restrictions on the sale of alcohol. Due to all these regulations and policy practices, Sweden has the second-highest rate on the alcohol-policy scales of the twenty-eight countries; it is only surpassed by Norway (Karlsson et al. 2012).

The regulation for tobacco is not as strict as it is for alcohol; in fact, Sweden rates just one point above the mid-point on the tobacco-control scale. What stands out here is that Sweden is one of the few countries to take tobacco into account in its national strategy; tobacco is normally treated separately.

As for policies for illicit substances, penalties are not determined according to the legal classification of substances. The government has not decriminalized drug possession, and harm-reduction policies are as strong is in the first model. Furthermore, although Sweden has aimed to export its policy approach, it has not obtained top-ranked EMCDDA best practices.

In this respect, Sweden's move towards a more 'well-being and relational management' strategy requires less strictness—one of the characteristics that has brought this country international recognition and which, so far, has proved useful for maintaining low levels of addictive substance consumption. This would imply the introduction of more prevention and harm-reduction policies.

To coordinate drug-related policies, in 2007 the Swedish government established an ad hoc body, 'Alcohol, Narcotic Drugs, Doping, and Tobacco'. This body advises the government and provides information through research, including a working group on coordinating the policy in the various ministerial subdivisions. Sweden implements drug-related policies through twenty-one counties, 290 municipalities, and local NGOs. The Swedish National Institute of Public Health—a state agency under the Ministry of Health—coordinates the counties and municipalities and their implementation of the action plans. This decentralization is also supported by county administrative boards, which are responsible for the supervision and distribution of financial support for drug policy interventions throughout the municipalities, and regional coordinators, who work on drugs and alcohol prevention within communities.

The same organizational structure characterizes the role of the Swedish National Board of Health and Welfare, which supports the implementation of the action plans. It works under the umbrella of the national government to select and fund non-profit organizations and businesses to implement treatment policies.

5.3 **Finland**

Like its Nordic counterparts, Finland obtains high rates in OECD quality of life and material living conditions (see Annex 13). More specifically, it is among the four countries that, on average, score more than eight out of ten in quality of life (OECD 2011b) and in sustainable governance indicators.

Although Finland did not start legislating drugs until 1994, only one year before its entrance into the EU, it is currently embracing a long-term approach, focusing on demand and supply, and promoting cooperation with different stakeholders. More specifically, the 2008–2011 government resolution has the following action guidelines coordinated by the Ministry of Social Affairs and Health (Government of Finland 2008):

1 Prevention and early intervention.

2 Fight against drug-related crime.

3 Treatment and harm reduction.

4 Penalties.

5 International cooperation.

6 Information and research on drug-related problems.

7 Drug policies coordination.

Finland is one of the few countries that not only decriminalize drug possession and use, but also implement severe regulation with strict policy control on tobacco and alcohol. Despite this holistic view, Finnish drug classification does not determine the final penalties. Moreover, it foresees prevention measures linked to mental health but has three types of prevention (universal, selective, and indicated) mainly implemented by NGOs. Harm reduction is also performed in treatment centres, while outreach and peer work are emerging to provide services to socially excluded drug consumers.

Alcohol policies in Finland have changed and become more liberalized since the country entered the EU. However, the government still retains power and control over alcohol through the state monopoly (Alko) on off-licence retail sales of alcoholic beverages with more than 4.7 per cent of alcohol. Alko Inc., founded in 1932, is an independent limited company wholly owned by the Finnish government and administered and supervised by the Ministry of Social Affairs and Health. The main intention of the Finnish Alcohol Act (Finnish Ministry of Social Affairs and Health 1994) is to avoid the negative effects on society and health that result from alcohol consumption.

Following regulation of the legal substances model and EU trends, Finland has an ad hoc coordinator body, the Drug Policy Co-ordination Group, which monitors the drug situation in Finland and supervises the implementation of cross-sectoral drug programmes in the public sector. Since many ministries, apart from Health and Social Affairs, are involved in decision-making and policy implementation, one of the group's key tasks is to coordinate the measures of the various administrative departments. While policy planning is decided at national level, the implementation process is led by the municipalities, ensuring the equal provision of vital social and health care services to all Finns. Provision and treatment implementation is the responsibility of the municipalities, which deliver these services through collaboration with NGOs and publicly funded foundations. Finnish facilities normally include treatment for both legal and illicit substances.

Finland implements one of the strictest policies on alcohol, only surpassed by Sweden and Norway (Karlsson et al. 2012). Finland, like most Nordic countries, has been deeply influenced by the temperance movement, and alcohol restrictions are not just government initiatives; they are also the result of public demand. A study conducted by Helsingin Sanomat (2010) reveals that nearly 70 per cent of Finns would reduce the blood alcohol content (BAC) threshold for drunk-driving cases.

Although Finland only rates two points above the tobacco scale mid-point, Finnish non-profit organizations, jointly with some businesses and experts in the medical field, have launched an innovative and unusual policy in order to pressure the government to take the necessary steps to eradicate tobacco consumption by 2040 (see Box 5.2). These policies on legal substances seem to have worked so far, since the country reports very low levels of tobacco and alcohol consumption. On the other hand, Finland does not seem to have a consumption problem related to illicit substances (cannabis and heroin), as its levels of consumption are below the EU average.

Finland is an exceptional case, presenting a set of indicators aimed at evaluating and monitoring policies. They include drug consumption indicators by age

---

Box 5.2: Finland: tobacco-free by 2040

This initiative, launched by fifteen non-profit and private organizations in the health field, urges the government of Finland to undertake policies aimed at making Finland a tobacco-free country by 2040. This would mean a 10 per cent reduction of tobacco use annually.

Source: data from Savutonsuomi website, available at www.savutonsuomi.fi/en.php, Copyright © 2012 Savuton Suomi*

---

groups and by addictive substance; the number of problematic drug consumers; periods of hospitalization; drug-related and infectious diseases; the seizure of illicit substances; and drug-related crimes.

5.4 **France**

French socio-economic indicators exceed the EU average and France performs well in the various OECD indicators. However, comparison with the Nordic countries reveals that France has the lowest rates in most of the OECD Better Life Initiative indicators as well as in sustainable governance indicators (see Annex 14). The main French policy lines focus on prevention, treatment, and fighting drugs (French Inter-departmental Mission for the Fight against Drugs and Drug Addiction 2008). Prevention measures deal mainly with illicit substances and alcohol. Nevertheless, France has played a pioneering role in placing both alcohol and illicit substances under the same umbrella, introducing this policy shift in its second strategy (1999–2002). The measures presented in the 2008–2011 French national strategy aim to prevent the use and the abuse of substances by raising awareness of drug-related laws and the risks associated with experimenting with drugs. One of the goals of these policies is to delay people's initial experimentation with drugs, implemented through universal prevention policies coordinated by the Ministry of Education.

Although supply reduction measures are not a top priority in France—as they are in Ireland and the UK—France has enhanced anti-drug-trafficking policies, implementing tougher economic penalties for traffickers, and has boosted international cooperation in order to reduce the entry of illicit substances into the country. The main reason for this policy is that France is both a transit and a final destination for illicit substances, and 'its narcotics market is particularly dynamic' (France—EMCDDA and OFDT National Report 2011: 9). This makes it necessary to tackle the supply side. Although the Ministry of Health is responsible for drug-related policies, the role of the Ministry of Interior is significant.

France criminalizes possession and use of illicit substances. Without distinguishing between possession for personal use or for commercialization, it does not differentiate penalties based on the risk posed by the substance. France's security-oriented approach is reinforced by the fact that the penalty for drug trafficking, when accompanied with aggravating circumstances, can be life imprisonment.

In summary, prevention is still the top priority of the French authorities when tackling legal and illicit substances. Although its policies are coordinated by the MILDT (Inter-ministerial Mission for the Fight against Drugs and Drug Addiction), the role of the Ministry of Education is also relevant in providing a universal prevention policy for primary and secondary schools. Treatment, on the other hand, is delivered by regional and local authorities.

Notwithstanding these measures, the French 2008–2011 strategy integrates harm-reduction policies 'intended to prevent transmission of infections, death from overdose by intravenous injection of drugs and social and psychological damage linked to drug addiction by substances classified as drugs' (France—EMCDDA Country Overview 2011). Examples for heroin consumers include a network of 135 low-threshold publicly funded agencies that provide syringe exchange programmes and the dispensing machines and pharmacies that sell state-subsidized sterikits (in 2008, 5.5 million sterikits were sold in France).

In 1991 France passed the *Loi Évin*, which became the foundation of the country's alcohol and tobacco policy. The *Loi Évin* is notable for its regulation of alcohol and tobacco advertisements (see Box 5.3). In spite of all these regulations, France ranks fourth—after Norway, Sweden, and Finland—on the alcohol policy scale. However, and in contrast to its Nordic counterparts, France's levels of alcohol consumption are still two percentage points above the mean for the twenty-eight. This can be explained by its being a wine-producing country and its different consumption patterns (more regular but less consumption of alcohol).

While harm-reduction and substitution treatments are available in France, most effort is directed towards supply reduction. With its combination of harm-reduction policies, introduced in 2004, we consider France to be becoming a public-health oriented country. Since 1982 France has had an ad hoc body for addictions. The MILDT plans and coordinates all public polices related to drugs, whether legal or illicit.

Although France is a centralized state, the French regions also play a part in policy implementation. Each region has a territorial project manager to avoid inconsistencies across territories. These project managers are required to plan multi-annual regional strategies aligned with the national strategy. The

---

Box 5.3: The *Loi Évin*

This French law forbids alcohol and tobacco advertising on television, in cinemas, and at sporting events. The only publicity permitted in France is through print media and display on billboards, with statutory restrictions. Alcohol advertisements can only refer to product characteristics, such as ingredients and origin, and all have to include health-warning labels.

Source: data from Loi Évin, *Loi no 91–32 du 10 janvier 1991 relative à la lutte contre le tabagisme et l'alcoolisme*, Copyright © 1991.

---

regional strategies are accompanied by annual action plans that take three aspects into account: prevention and treatment, implementation of the law, and action against trafficking.

5.5 Ireland

Ireland has the highest unemployment rate among the countries that follow this second model, and has been deeply affected by the economic crisis. In November 2010 Ireland was bailed out by the troika of the European Union, the European Central Bank, and the International Monetary Fund. However, it still scores the EU average in the different OECD Better Life Initiative variables, as well as the status and management index (Sustainable Governance Indicators 2011). According to the Inglehart World Values Survey (2012), Ireland is the only country in this cluster with traditional rather than rational values. In this sense, Inglehart and Welzel (2010) classify Ireland jointly with the UK, although Irish citizens tend to be more conservative and traditionalist than their British neighbours (see Annex 18).

Ireland is one of the very few countries that makes supply reduction a top priority in its national strategy. However, Ireland not only has strict policies towards legal substances (like all countries in this model), but it also decriminalizes drug possession. This implies that the country tolerates drug consumption as a reality and assumes that prohibiting possession will not solve the problem. As noted in Chapter 2, countries that decriminalize drug possession also tend to embrace more harm-reduction policies. In fact, Ireland goes one step further and establishes penalties for illicit substances according to drug classification and taking into account the associated risks.

Ireland's national drug strategy (2009–2016) focuses on the harm drugs cause to individuals and society through five pillars: supply reduction, prevention, treatment, rehabilitation, and research. These are linked to the following five strategic objectives:

1 A safer society through supply reduction.

2 Reducing problematic drug consumption across society as a whole.

3 Providing treatment, rehabilitation, and harm-reduction services according to each drug user's need.

4 Provision of necessary and precise data about the magnitude and nature of substance abuse and consumption in Ireland.

5 Provision of an efficient framework to implement the national strategy.

Ireland still has an official alcohol prevention policy (Österberg and Karlsson 2003), with regulations governing retail sales of alcoholic beverages and licences required to operate off- and on-premise retail outlets. The country has also introduced liberal free-market policies leading to the deregulation of alcohol licences, reductions in excise duty, the removal of price controls, and the self-regulation of sales outlets and advertising bodies. Hence alcohol policies focus on encouraging individual responsibility through health-promotion and harm-reduction initiatives (Alcohol Abuse Among Adolescents in Europe 2012). Despite these measures, Ireland still ranks high on the EU alcohol policy scale (see Fig. 5.3).

Ireland is a notably fertile ground for tobacco smuggling (Retailers Against Smuggling 2012). The tobacco industry claims it loses more than €800 million in turnover every year through smuggling. One of the main goals of Irish tobacco control is to reduce the number of cigarettes consumed on which duty is not paid. In this kind of case, the interests of government and industry might be more aligned, since the former aims to avoid tax leakage while the latter aims to retain its market share. The high prices imposed on tobacco are reflected in the tobacco scale, which, jointly with the UK, is the highest among the twenty-eight.

Despite developing a strategy focused on illicit substances, since 2012 the Irish government has taken steps towards a more comprehensive approach for dealing with illicit substances and alcohol. Notwithstanding the involvement of the Ministry of State, the Department of Health is the institution responsible for the day-to-day operational coordination of drug policy (Ireland—EMCDDA Country Overview 2011). Ireland gives the ultimate responsibility to the Ministry of Health, and involves non-profit organizations in decision-making but excludes businesses from the process. Following the European trend, Ireland has an ad hoc coordinating body for addiction policies, the Oversight Forum on Drugs, which monitors and examines the progress of the strategy and addresses any operational difficulty related to policy implementation. Chaired by the Department of Health and the Minister of State, the Oversight Forum on Drugs also includes representatives from the bodies responsible for implementing the national drugs strategy, government departments, state agencies, and community and voluntary sectors.

Apart from this body, there are also two units under the Department of Health tasked with the day-to-day operational coordination of drug policy: the Drug Policy Unit and the Drugs Programme Unit. The former oversees the implementation of the national strategy and the latter manages the projects implemented by local and regional drugs task forces, which are part of the Drugs Initiative Programme.

Although Ireland does not decentralize policy-making, the role of the regions throughout the implementation process is very relevant. Ireland has established a mechanism to promote the participation of local communities as well as non-profit organizations at different stages of its drug and addiction policies. In this respect, Ireland has established local and regional drugs task forces, which are mainly involved in the coordination of local services. It is worth noting that each task force agrees its own action plan.

Finally, the National Advisory Committee on Drugs conducts, commissions, and analyses research across the areas of prevalence, prevention, consequences, and treatment. Grouping officials, communities, volunteers from non-profit organizations, and researchers, this advisory committee assists the government on drug-policy issues. Its ultimate aim is to improve knowledge and understanding of drug-related problems, provide the government with timely data and research, and disseminate findings.

5.6 **The UK**

The UK performs well in socio-economic indicators such as GDP and in the OECD Better Life Initiative indicators, obtaining on average 7.24 out of 10 (see Annex 33). The few indicators in which the UK performs poorly are related to inequality (Eurostat 2011b); among the countries in the regulation of legal substances model it performs worst in the at-risk poverty rate after social transfer.

In contrast to the rest of the countries in this model, the UK places responsibility for addictions exclusively under the Home Office (rather than the Ministry of Health). The main body in the field of drugs in the UK is the Advisory Council on the Misuse of Drugs (ACMD), an advisory public body of the Home Office. Established in 1971 under the Misuse of Drugs Act, the ACMD produces reports based on in-depth inquiries and makes recommendations to the government on the 'control of dangerous and harmful drugs, including classification and scheduling under the Misuse of Drugs Act 1971 and its regulations' (Advisory Council on the Misuse of Drugs 2012). This country still embraces some safety and disease approach characteristics, for example making supply reduction a priority of the national strategy.

Notwithstanding, the motto of the 2010 national strategy is indicative: 'Reducing demand, restricting supply, building recovery: supporting people to live a drug-free life'. In contrast to the UK's former strategy, the 2010 strategy is much more focused on rehabilitation than on harm reduction: 'instead of focusing primarily on reducing the harms caused by drug misuse, our approach will be to go much further and offer every support for people to choose recovery as an achievable way out of dependency' (UK Drug Strategy 2010: 2).

This strategy is mainly focused on prevention and, as noted by the EMCDDA (United Kingdom—EMCDDA Country Overview 2011), it establishes a whole-life approach to drug prevention, from early age to families, and there are universal, selective, and indicated prevention policies. The relevance of prevention policies is confirmed by the fact that the UK has two top-rated best practices in prevention (EMCDDA 2011c). Another interesting point of this strategy, broadly shared by most of the countries within this model, is that it includes alcohol use, thus taking into account legal and illicit substances.

It is in the UK's means of tackling licit substances that we can see clear commonalities with the Nordic countries and France. There is a strict regulative and

---

Box 5.4: The UK government's U-turn on a minimum price per unit of alcohol

In November 2012 the UK government designated a minimum price per unit of alcohol. Minimum unit pricing is a method to tackle excessive alcohol consumption by reducing its affordability. This method makes it 'illegal to sell alcohol below a set price per unit, and the policy is intended especially to tackle the problem of cheap alcohol from supermarkets and off-licensed outlets' (Institute of Alcohol Studies 2013). In parallel with the minimum unit price, the UK government was also considering introducing a 'ban on discounted multi-buy alcohol promotions in supermarkets' (Institute of Alcohol Studies 2013). But in July 2013 the government backtracked, claiming, 'this will remain a policy under consideration but will not be taken forward at this time. We do not yet have enough concrete evidence that its introduction would be effective in reducing harms associated with problem drinking, without penalising people who drink responsibly' (Paskin 2013).

Source: data from Paskin, B., *UK government scraps minimum pricing plans*, The Spirits Business [online journal], Copyright © 2013, available from http://www.thespiritsbusiness.com/2013/07/uk-government-scraps-minimum-pricing-plans/ and Institute of Alcohol Studies, Government U-turn on minimum unit pricing of alcohol in England, *The Globe*, Volume 3, pp. 8–9, Copyright © 2013.

evidence-based approach to reducing alcohol and tobacco consumption, such as the price of alcohol beverages (17 points above the EU average), which allows us to establish links with patterns of drinking in the Nordic countries. The UK failed in 2013 in implementing innovative measures for alcohol, which were characterized by increasing the regulative pressure on alcoholic beverages (see Box 5.4).

The UK is among the countries that devolve policy-making to decentralized structures, more specifically to Wales, Scotland, and Northern Ireland. These countries of the UK can develop their own policies for drugs and addiction. Each has passed its own strategy, such as the Road to Recovery: A New Approach to Tackling Scotland's Drug Problem, and Working Together to Reduce Harm: The Substance Misuse Strategy for Wales 2008–2018.

5.7 **Norway**

Norway is the only country included in this study that is not part of the EU. Its welfare state model and its OECD Better Life Initiative indicators are similar to Sweden and Finland; it rates among the top five in most of them (see Annex 25). Furthermore, it has one of the highest GDP per capita of countries within this model (181; EU = 100). It has the lowest GINI index among the 28 (22.9; average 29.3), and the lowest unemployment rate (3.3 per cent).

Despite not having a national strategy, the Norwegian action plan is halfway between a strategy and a plan. The overriding goal of the action plan for 2008–2012 was to reduce the negative consequences of drug and alcohol use for individuals and society as a whole. Hence, much like Sweden, Norway not only tackles legal and illicit substances together, but also attends to the consequences that addictive substances can cause for society in general. The action plan has five main objectives (Norwegian Ministry of Health and Care Services 2007):

1 A clear public-health perspective.

2 Better quality and increased competence in the implementation of the policy.

3 More accessible services and greater social inclusion.

4 More binding cooperation between actors implementing the policy.

5 Increased user influence and greater attention to the interests of children and family members.

Like other countries in this model, apart from the UK, the Ministry of Health and Care Services has overall responsibility for drugs and alcohol policies and for coordinating efforts involving several sectors. Although it has not decriminalized drug possession or use, Norway has innovative policy practices in the field of harm reduction, including drug injection rooms in Oslo since 2004. Norway's priority is harm reduction and these policies are widely extended throughout the country. The Norwegian drug policy has a specific coordinating organism, the Stoltenberg Committee, tasked with assessing how drug addicts and alcoholics most in need can receive better help.

According to alcohol policy scales (Karlsson et al. 2012), the Norwegian alcohol policy is the most restrictive and regulative in Europe. The policy was implemented in the twentieth century, and its uninterrupted longevity has been possible thanks to a consensus among political parties, whose main objective has been to minimize social and health problems related to alcohol consumption. Policies governing legal substances intend to reduce harm by reducing availability. The main tools that accomplish this are an alcohol monopoly, a local licensing system, and high excise on alcohol. Norway also has the highest EU excise on tobacco, which translates into high levels of alcohol and tobacco smuggling from Denmark and Sweden.

Broadly, policy planning in the field of addictions in Norway is the responsibility of the national government, while implementation is coordinated by municipalities, which have sufficient leeway to decide on specific issues, such as whether or not to establish injection rooms. Finally, universal prevention programmes are established and administered by municipalities jointly with NGOs.

5.8 Conclusion to Model 2 in Europe

Once again, this model brings together countries with different welfare-state traditions. More specifically, we find Nordic, Anglo-Saxon, and continental countries (Esping-Andersen 1990). Notwithstanding, their levels of GDP per capita, income, and OECD Better Life Initiative variables are above the mean for the twenty-eight. The most significant divergence regarding contextual measures is that related to inequality indicators measured through at-risk poverty rate after social transfer (Eurostat 2011a, 2011b); both show that the Anglo-Saxon countries have higher levels of inequality than the Nordic countries, which are widely known for their universalist welfare state.

The distinctive features of these countries are a regulatory approach to licit substances and loose measures to combat illicit substances. These countries have prioritized policies aimed at tackling legal substances over policies towards illicit substances. This strict regulation is explained when we analyse alcohol consumption, especially the heavy consumption of distilled beverages, and the harm this causes to society as well as to individual health.

In this respect, model 2 groups the six countries of the sample that implement evidence-based regulation on alcohol and tobacco. Although their approaches are quite different—the Nordic countries control alcohol consumption through monopolies, and the UK, Ireland, and France do it through regulation—the final objective is to reduce the level of alcohol and tobacco consumption, improve quality of life, and reduce the rate of deaths attributable to the consumption of legal substances.

It is worth noting here that the Nordic and Anglo-Saxon countries are pioneers in evidence-based research. However, only one of these countries—the UK—is implementing best practices with the highest rate granted by the EMCDDA. Compared with the countries in the first model, the countries within this model do not implement as many innovative policies and are not as proactive.

All the countries in this model have been classified as having a comprehensive policy-making structure; they tend to tackle legal and illicit substances together, involve non-profit organizations in decision-making processes, have an ad hoc body, decentralize implementation, and have a long trajectory in legislating illicit substances.

Chapter 6

Model 3: Transitioning (Austria, Bulgaria, Cyprus, Denmark, Poland, Slovenia)

6.1 Description of the model: Approaches to the governance of addictions

This is the most divergent of the four clusters obtained through our quantitative analysis. First, it includes continental and Nordic welfare state regimes plus Cyprus and Slovenia, which, according to the frame taken into account (see Chapter 2), were not classified in any of the four welfare state regimes (Esping-Andersen 1990). However, the most outstanding differences within this model are those related to contextual data. Within this model we can find the country with the lowest rate in GDP per capita and income level of our sample, Bulgaria, together with Austria and Denmark, which are among the top ten in both indicators and perform very well in economic and non-material domains, according to the OECD (2011b). Furthermore, Bulgaria and Cyprus are not OECD member states. It is also worth noting that Cyprus, Poland, and Bulgaria in particular have higher levels of inequality than Austria, Denmark, and Slovenia (Eurostat 2011b). Regarding Inglehart's World Values Survey (2012), the majority of the countries are classified within the Catholic Europe group. The only exceptions are Cyprus, which is not classified in any group, and Bulgaria, which is regarded as an ex-Communist country. Its citizens thus tend to have survival rather than self-expression values, which emphasize physical security and report low levels of trust and tolerance.

Levels of consumption of legal substances in these countries are above the average for the twenty-eight, except for Cyprus, which rates way below the mean not only for the consumption of legal substances but also for illicit substances (see Figs 4.1, 4.2, 5.1, and 5.2). While it is difficult to identify a cross-cutting trend in the strategies of these countries, they appear to have a safety and disease strategy rather than a well-being and relational management approach. We note that most of these countries are closer to having a comprehensive structure to deal with addictions. This is a cluster of countries transitioning from a traditional to a more comprehensive model, with few exceptions (see Box 6.1).

> ## Box 6.1: Key elements of the transitioning model
>
> – It is closer to the safety and disease strategy than to the well-being and relational management approach.
> – Treatment rather than punishment.
> – High levels of consumption of legal substances.
> – Most of the countries are shifting their policies and embracing well-being and relational management measures, such as best practices and evidence-based regulation for alcohol.
> – None of the countries decriminalizes possession.
> – Low ranking in tobacco scales.
> – Substance separation approach.
> – Decentralization in policy making.
> – A cluster of countries transitioning from one model to another, especially from the traditional to a more comprehensive model.

None of the countries in this model decriminalizes possession. All of them make the Ministry of Health responsible for addiction, and prioritize treatment and prevention issues over supply reduction. They do not have injection rooms as a harm-reduction policy and the tobacco control scale in every country in this model is below the mid-point (Joossens and Raw 2010).

This is the only model in which none of the countries tackles legal and illicit substances together or involves non-profit or private organizations in the decision-making process. Moreover, most of them decentralize policy-making and implementation.

6.2 **Poland**

The Polish drug law implements the 'treat rather than punish principle' (Poland—EMCDDA Country Overview 2011). In this respect, Poland has a more well-being and relational management strategy than other countries in this model. There are two key indicators that align Poland with a well-being and relational management approach (see Annex 26); on the one hand, it rates above the mean for the twenty-eight in alcohol policy scales, while on the other, it is the only country following model 3 that has top-rated EMCDDA best practices (see Box 6.2).

Box 6.2: Polish best practices in prevention

Fantastyczne Mozliwosci and Program Domowych Detektywow

Both these best practices are based on US programmes—Amazing Alternatives and the Slick Tracy Home Team Programme, respectively. They aim to prevent drinking among adolescents aged 11–13. *Fantastyczne Mozliwosci* consists of six teacher/peer-led classroom sessions combined with parent-child activities to be undertaken at home.

Source: data from European Monitoring Centre for Drugs and Drug Addiction (EMCDDA), *Best Practice Portal*, available from http://www.emcdda.europa.eu/best-practice, Copyright © EMCDDA, 1995–2012.

The main objective of the Polish national strategy is to reduce drug consumption in society; hence, it is more focused on demand reduction and more specifically on prevention, which is the principal aim of the strategy. Its national strategy for 2011–2016 specifies the following areas of action (Polish Government 2011):

1 Prevention

2 Treatment, rehabilitation, harm reduction, and social reintegration

3 Supply reduction

4 International cooperation

5 Research and monitoring.

As noted, Poland rates the fifth highest score on the alcohol policy scale (after Norway, Sweden, Finland, and France), because of its production licences, control of on- and off-licence sales, strict control on age limits, low levels of BAC, and restrictive policy towards alcohol advertising and marketing. Notwithstanding, the levels of unrecorded consumption are still above the mean for the twenty-eight, giving Poland one of the highest differences between recorded and unrecorded consumption, comparable only to the Eastern European countries grouped in the traditional model.

Furthermore, Poland is not as tough on drug crime as other CEECs. Polish punishments for possessing and trafficking drugs are aligned to the EU recommendations, and never exceed ten years' imprisonment. Despite not making a legal distinction between drug dealers and user-dealers, when someone sells drugs in order to fund an addiction the offence may be considered of lesser gravity. Although Poland does not have injection rooms, it has implemented harm-reduction policies since 1989. More specifically, it has provided needle and syringe exchange programmes and prevention-related educational programmes.

Like the other countries in this model, Poland tackles legal and illicit substances separately and does not involve non-profit and private organizations in decision-making. It also has an ad hoc advisory body that coordinates drug and addiction policies, the Council for Counteracting Drug Addiction, created in 2001. This body coordinates state policy actions, monitors the implementation of the national strategy, and boosts inter-ministerial and cross-sectoral cooperation. Meanwhile, the National Bureau of Drug prevention, under the Ministry of Health, commissions and conducts drug-related research and develops preventive programmes to be delivered in schools, in cooperation with the Ministry of Education and the Ministry of the Interior.

Prevention is mainly organized and coordinated by the National Bureau for Drug Prevention and the State Agency for Prevention of Alcohol-related Problems. However, at regional and local levels the responsibility for drug prevention and implementation of drug treatment lies with provincial and local government. These policies are delivered through a wide range of providers, mainly NGOs that have signed a contractual agreement with the National Health Fund.

6.3 **Austria**

Within model 3, Austria has the highest GDP per capita and lowest levels of unemployment (see Annex 6). Moreover, it has high scores in the OECD Better Life Initiative variables, sustainable governance indicators, and inequality indexes (Eurostat 2011a, 2011b).

Austria's main objective is to have a society as free from addictions as possible. More specifically, the government advocates the principle of 'treatment instead of punishment'. To achieve this, Austrian policy is split into four pillars: prevention, advice and treatment, social integration, and quality assurance and documentation. Austria still criminalizes both drug use and drug possession, and drug classification does not determine final penalties.

The lack of a national strategy or action plan has made the Narcotic Substances Act (*Suchtmittelgesetz*—SMG), approved in 1998, the main framework of Austria's drug policy at national level. In 2014 the Austrian government is expected to pass the first national strategy built on evidence-based research and on a broad definition of prevention, taking into account both drug use and different forms of addiction not related to specific substances (addictive behaviours), and then a political adoption is necessary. Interestingly, the SMG gives more relevance to the quantity than to the kind of substance carried by individuals; the only exception in this respect is cannabis, which is subject to special provisions and allows the individual carrying it a wide range of alternatives to punishment. Moreover, Austria distinguishes between the addict and the trafficker, imposing different penalties on each.

Austria still adopts a safety and disease strategy towards drugs and addictions rather than a well-being and relational management approach. It does not determine penalties according to drug classification; it does not decriminalize possession; it does not have injection rooms; it rates very low in the tobacco and alcohol scales; and it has no top-rated practices recognized by the EMCDDA.

If we look at illicit substances, the overall picture confirms this diagnosis. Austria has higher penalties than the EU recommendations for trafficking, including life imprisonment as an option for those who are caught trafficking illicit substances. On the other hand, penalties for drug possession are below the EU recommendations, but incur a minimum of three years' imprisonment. Austrian safety and disease strategy is reinforced by the fact that none of the provincial governments has decriminalized drug possession, although some do consider drug use a civil rather than a criminal offence. Regarding harm reduction, which is considered a pillar of the public-health approach, most of the measures are oriented towards 'low-threshold assistance and to reducing the risk of problematic consequence of drug use' (Austria—EMCDDA Country Overview 2011). These low-threshold services, jointly with outpatient drug services, syringe-vending machines, and pharmacies, have been determinants of the implementation of syringe exchange programmes.

The loose regulation through which Austria controls legal substances merits a special mention. Austria has the lowest EU rate on the tobacco control scale (Joossens and Raw 2010). The price of alcoholic beverages in Austria is below the mean for the twenty-eight; there is no legal requirement for a licence to produce, sell, or distribute alcohol, and there are no restrictions on places and times at which alcohol can be sold. These are some of the main reasons why Austria rates only two places above the bottom of the alcohol policy scale—the countries with lower rates are Malta and Luxembourg (Karlsson et al. 2012). The Austrian government has traditionally had a weak position on tobacco control. In 1997 Austria and Germany jointly voted against the EU directive on tobacco advertising (Joossens and Raw 2007).

Austria tackles drugs and addictive substances through the Ministry of Health, more specifically through the Federal Drug Coordination Office (FDCO) and *Bundesdrogenforum* (Federal Drug Forum, or FDF). The FDCO is responsible for the operational coordination of federal drug policies, the preparation of ministerial decisions in the field, and the representation of Austria at

European and international level. This office has three members, one from the Ministry of Health and two from the Ministry of the Interior and the Ministry of Justice (representatives from other ministries can also be invited on an ad hoc basis). The FDF consists of the nine federal drug coordinators, representatives from federal ministries and local government, experts, and scientists. Its main goal is to provide sound advice to the Minister of Health.

Austria is a federal country, and the Austrian states play an important role in the processes of policy-making, implementation, and evaluation of drug and addiction measures. In contrast to Austria's central government, each of the nine states (Vorarlberg, Tyrol, Carinthia, Salzburg, Styria, Upper Austria, Lower Austria, Vienna, and Burgenland) has its own drug strategy or action plan, and appoints its own drug and addiction coordinators, who have the responsibility of managing addiction policies. Although the drug coordinators' tasks can differ for each state, in most cases they are responsible for planning and implementing drug policy measures. The nine coordinators have their own forum for discussion and coordination, the Provincial Conference of Drug Coordinators, which produces joint statements and common positions.

The main policy lines in Austria, prevention and treatment, are mainly organized and implemented by each individual state and local government under the guidance of state coordinators. Prevention is generally focused on preventing addiction to legal substances and is mainly settled and implemented by local and state institutions under the direction of state addiction prevention units. The addiction prevention forums of Salzburg and Vienna and the state coordination and control bodies also play a role in these processes. Interestingly, prevention policies at school level try to involve as many stakeholders in the school community as possible, as well as regional addiction experts, which reinforces the comprehensive structure of this country. Like prevention, treatment is coordinated and funded by each of the nine Austrian states, social insurance, and the federal government. Again, regional public institutions and NGOs are the major actors in the delivery of drug-related treatment. It is worth mentioning here that substitution treatment is widely available and has become the most important form of treatment in Austria.

6.4 **Bulgaria**

Bulgaria is the EU member state with the lowest GDP per capita and the lowest level of income (see Annex 8). The country is regarded as the gateway to the EU for heroin produced in Central and South-East Asia. This has a direct impact on Bulgaria's approach to dealing with illicit substances and has also made heroin the illicit drug most associated with problematic consumption.

Bulgaria's drug strategy is clearly aligned with a safety and disease approach. It is one of the few countries that makes supply reduction one of the top priorities of its national strategy. More specifically, the national anti-drug strategy for 2009–2013 has two main objectives:

1 Protect public health and citizens' well-being, guaranteeing high levels of security through the adoption of a balanced and integrated approach towards drug problems.

2 Reduce the supply of illicit substances while increasing the efficiency of the law and intensifying preventive measures against crime and drugs.

Bulgaria's main goals are to protect the health and the well-being of its citizens, safeguard a high level of security, and reduce the supply of drugs and precursor chemicals. Apart from this, Bulgaria mainly undertakes prevention and treatment policies, while those related to harm reduction are a residual part of its strategic approach.

It is worth noting that Bulgaria and Malta are the only countries in this model to introduce well-being in their national strategy. This is a characteristic that should be aligned with a well-being and relational management strategy but in Bulgaria's case it is not sufficiently supported by other policies, such as harm reduction, decriminalization, and regulation. In fact, as we show in Chapter 2, including well-being and public health in the aims of the national strategy is negatively associated with having a 'well-being and relational management' strategy. This is because countries with these characteristics normally rate poorly in the rest of the items taken into account.

Bulgaria's safety and disease strategy is reinforced by the strict sanctions it implements for the use, possession and trafficking of drugs, and criminal organization—in all the cases above the EU recommendations (Council of the EU 2004bb). This can be explained by the country's geostrategic location, which makes it a transhipment country for South-East Asian heroin entering the European market (CIA 2012). Another example of Bulgarian 'safety and disease' strategy can be found in its penal code, which states that 'a person who without due permit manufactures, processes, acquires, distributes, stores, keeps, transports or carries narcotic drugs or analogues thereof, shall be punished, for high risk narcotic drugs—by imprisonment of 10 to 15 years and a fine, and for low risk narcotic drugs—by imprisonment of three to 15 years' (Article 354a).

Finally, regarding legal substances, Bulgaria rates very low on both alcohol and tobacco scales, which means that it can still impose stricter regulations aimed at reducing the accessibility and consumption of legal substances. In fact, as noted by Joossens and Raw (2010), prices in Bulgaria increased between 2007 and 2010 only because of the 2002/10/EC Tobacco Tax Directive.

The National Drugs Council, established in 2001, is a body of the Council of Ministers of the Republic of Bulgaria, chaired by the Minister of Health, and operates at inter-ministerial level. It is responsible for the implementation and coordination of policy against the abuse of drugs and drug trafficking.

Treatment is provided by public, non-profit, and private organizations, depending on the policy, and is mainly focused on substitution treatment for opioid users. Harm-reduction policies are still uncommon and are provided by NGOs, which target at-risk groups and provide services such as needle and syringe exchanges, and information on safe injection, overdose, and infectious diseases.

6.5 **Cyprus**

Cyprus understands addictions as an issue that is not only 'linked to biological degradation, but that also leads to marginalization, criminal offences, organized crime and thereby creates an imperative for social participation and a horizontal approach' (Cyprus National Strategy on Drugs 2009: 5). The national strategy also recognizes that addiction problems are political, social, cultural, and moral challenges. The strategy can be regarded as being closer to a safety and disease approach, although it increasingly promotes alternative measures to imprisonment for those committing certain drug-related crimes. The EMCDDA (Cyprus—EMCDDA Country Overview 2011) notes, 'there has been a tendency towards increased sentencing in recent years, there is also an on-going effort to promote the implementation of alternative measures to imprisonment in the criminal justice system'.

The ministries of Health and Education develop and coordinate policies in the field of addictions, while the Cyprus Anti-Drugs Council (CAC) is the authority responsible for coordinating actions related to drug policies. The CAC coordinates public institutions that provide treatment in cooperation with NGOs. It is chaired by the Ministry of Education; the vice-chair is the chairperson of the Cyprus Youth Board. Despite being administratively divided into six districts, these local administrations do not play relevant roles in addiction policies. This is mainly due to the size of the country.

The main priorities of the first Cypriot national strategy (2004–2009) were prevention and supply reduction; nonetheless, the structure was almost the same as the EU's strategy, with four main pillars: demand reduction, supply reduction, international cooperation, and information and evaluation. Cyprus embraced the main policy guidelines of the EU. The second Cypriot national strategy on drugs and addictions was passed in 2009. In contrast to many EU strategies, Cyprus avoids the traditional dichotomous approach based on demand and supply reduction, and its strategy embodies prevention, treatment, social integration, and harm reduction.

The Cypriot safety and disease approach is demonstrated in the seriousness of its legal sanctions. For instance, possessing heroin can be punished with up to twelve years' imprisonment, while the maximum sentence for trafficking either heroin or cannabis is imprisonment for life. Penalties for possession of less harmful substances (such as amphetamines and buprenorphine) are up to four years. In contrast to many EU countries, in Cyprus drug-related crimes are almost always brought to court. There are only two mitigating conditions for sanctions: (1) the drug offender is under 25 and the amount can be considered for personal use; (2) the drug offender is an addict. In spite of this strictness, Cyprus is an exception in this model because, like Denmark, drug classification determines the penalties imposed (see Annex 9).

6.6 **Denmark**

The Danish national strategy was approved in 2010 and is named the Fight Against Drugs II (the first was approved in 2003). It is based on four principles: prevention, treatment (including treatment in prisons), harm reduction, and control (including law enforcement). However, the Danish strategy is charac-terized by its strictness and its focus on the fight against drugs while striving for a drug-free society. Thus, though the focus is on prevention and treatment, harm-reduction policies are mainly pragmatic, sensible, and initiated in consideration of the weakest drug users and society in general.

Denmark's main institution responsible for coordinating drugs and addictions policy is the Ministry of Health and Prevention, although it collaborates with the ministries of Social Affairs, Justice, and Tax Affairs. Notwithstanding, until 2011, the main institution in charge was the Ministry of the Interior. From 1848 to 2007 the ministries of Health and the Interior were a single institution. This changed after the 2007 elections. Since 2011 the Ministry of Health and Prevention has been in charge of coordinating policies on drugs and addictions. This is a shift that should be interpreted as a movement towards a more well-being and relational management strategy.

Most of the policy-making on drugs and addictions is decided at national level by central government; however, the Danish municipalities are responsible for prevention, treatment, and the social reintegration of drug users. Thus, municipalities work closely with the Ministry of Health in monitoring drug use and developing appropriate responses. More specifically, municipalities have to plan universal and selective prevention in schools, communities, and local recreational centres. Furthermore, after the local government reform of 2007,

> ### Box 6.3: Danish alco-locks
>
> Similarly to Sweden, some bus and truck companies in Denmark are intro-ducing alco-locks. The alco-lock, or ignition lock, is a mechanism like a breathalyser, installed on a motor vehicle's dashboard. Before the vehicle can be started, the driver must exhale into the device. If the resultant breath-alcohol concentration is greater than the programmed blood-alcohol con-centration, the device prevents the engine from being started. Arriva, a bus company operating throughout Denmark, has installed alco-locks in their vehicles in order to ensure that bus drivers do not drink and drive.

municipalities became responsible for organizing the social and the medical treatment of drug users, while the regions are responsible for psychiatric care, and primary and public healthcare. The latest national strategy recognizes that drug abuse is a complex issue that requires the involvement of different institu-tions across professional and sector boundaries. This has led to the involvement of decentralized structures in policy-making and implementation processes.

The regulation and practices on legal substances in Denmark have been con-verging with that of its Nordic counterparts (see Box 6.3). Thus, although Den-mark still rates below the mean on the alcohol policy scale and scores less than the mid-point on the tobacco control scale (see Annex 11), recent legislation has enhanced the evidence-based regulation of this country. Since the 2000s Denmark's policy has shifted from a liberal to a more restrictive approach. Den-mark restricted off-licence sales of all alcoholic beverages, reduced the legal BAC, and established stricter rules on publicity and sponsorship. Until the 1998, when the government introduced a minimum age of 15, there was no age limit for the purchase of off-licence alcohol (Møller 2002). Between 2009 and 2011 the sale of alcohol was regulated through laws on prevention, treatment, advertising, marketing, licences, sales, and drink driving (Denmark—EMCD-DA Country Overview 2011).

Finally, Denmark stands out for its transparency and accountability. It is one of the few EU member states that explicitly presents a budget for addictions and drugs. The government specifies that €15 million will be allocated to accom-plish the objectives and projects defined in the 2010 national strategy.

6.7 Slovenia

Like the Czech Republic, Slovenia has traditionally been regarded as a special case among former communist countries. Slovenia was the richest part of the former Yugoslavia and its transition to a welfare capitalist model was very smooth, involving no armed conflict. Its socio-economic performance throughout the first decades of independence was very positive, and enabled Slovenia to become a member of the EU in 2004. A sign of this good performance is its average in the OECD Better Life Initiative (see Annex 30): 5.82 is very close to the mean of the OECD countries in this study. Although rating below the mean for the twenty-eight in GDP per capita and euros/inhabitant, Slovenia performs better than Portugal and the Czech Republic (both in model 1). Despite its status as a relatively new independent state, Slovenia has more than twenty years' experience in the field of harm reduction, although these kinds of policy are normally delivered by non-profit organizations funded by the Ministry for Labour, Family, and Social Affairs.

The Slovenian Resolution on the National Programme in the Field of Drugs for 2004–2009 (Slovenian Government 2004) only takes into account illicit substances and focuses on prevention, especially in schools, in order to deter and lower the numbers of young consumers. The pillars of this strategy are information systems, reducing the demand for drugs, preventing drug supply, synthetic drugs, accelerating international cooperation, coordination on various levels, research work, evaluation, and education. The top priority of universal prevention in Slovenia is developing and strengthening life skills, promoting healthy lifestyles, and establishing safe and stimulating environments.

Drug consumption in Slovenia is not an offence and illicit possession of drugs is considered a minor offence under the Production and Trade in Illicit Drugs Act. However, penalties for the trafficking and commercialization of illicit substances are above the EU recommendations. In 2011, the National Assembly of the Republic of Slovenia adopted an amendment to the penal code that provides that an action to facilitate illicit drug use is not punishable if it is in the context of a programme of drug addiction treatment or is a controlled use of drugs that conforms to the law approved and is implemented within the framework or under the supervision of public-health authorities (e.g. in a safe injecting room).

Slovenia reports higher alcohol consumption levels than the EU average. It does not require licences for producing or distributing alcoholic beverages; however, it mandates the use of ignition locks in certain cases. Despite being classified as an Eastern and Central Eastern European country (Anderson et al. 2012), Slovenian drinking patterns are similar to those observed in other Mediterranean countries, i.e. daily consumption during meals and the rejection of public drunkenness. However, in contrast to Mediterranean countries, Slovenia has developed a set of consistent evidence-based regulations, such as a total ban on the sale of alcoholic beverages at sport events and restrictions on times and places for off-licence sales.

Like every country in this transitioning model, Slovenia rates below the midpoint on the tobacco control scale. However, the 2007 Act on Limiting the Use of Tobacco Products aligned with the EU Directives—on the approximation of the laws, regulations, and administrative provisions of the member states relating to the advertising and sponsorship of tobacco products—increasing the regulation and severity of penalties for those breaking the law.

Slovenia has local action groups that develop and coordinate anti-drug policies at local level. Each group includes 'representatives from municipalities, kindergartens, schools, parents, youth, drug users, health centres, centres for social work, employment services, police, courts, non-governmental organizations, religious communities, media, and other interested members of the public' (Slovenia—EMCDDA Country Overview 2011). Thus, the Slovenian authorities introduce participation in addiction policies and promote the involvement of local stakeholders in the planning, monitoring, and coordinating stages of addiction policy.

6.8 Conclusion to Model 3 in Europe

The transitioning model is made up of the most divergent and most unexpected group of countries. As we noted at the beginning of this chapter, in it we find the country with the lowest rates in socio-economic indicators (Bulgaria) together with Denmark and Austria, which rank high in material and non-material variables.

The strategy of these countries is mainly characterized by making the Ministry of Health the main institution responsible for drugs and addictions policy and by prioritizing treatment, prevention, and harm reduction above supply reduction. Taking all this into account, we could say that these countries have been clustered together because of the *absence* of a set of characteristics: decriminalization of possession, injection rooms, tobacco-control scale, and public-health aims. These countries do not tackle legal and illicit substances together; hence, they focus on the substances rather than on addictions. Furthermore, few of the countries in this group involve non-profit and private organizations in the decision-making process.

The main characteristic of these countries is that they are transitioning from one model to another. More specifically, our conclusion is that most of the countries in model 3 are moving from the traditional model to a more comprehensive one (either the first or second of our models here) with few exceptions. Poland, Slovenia, Bulgaria, and Cyprus to some extent follow a model similar to the traditional one; however, they make the Ministry of Health the responsible institution and tend towards a well-being and relational management strategy.

Second, Austria appears to follow the first model more closely; however, it still has not decriminalized the possession of illicit substances. Finally, Denmark is normally associated with the regulation of legal substances model, but its regulatory approach is not as strict as that of its Nordic neighbours. Regarding the exceptions, Bulgaria and Cyprus seem to be more closely related to countries within the traditional approach model.

Chapter 7

Model 4: The traditional approach (Estonia, Greece, Hungary, Latvia, Lithuania, Malta, Romania, Slovakia)

7.1 Description of the model: Approaches to the governance of addictions

This model gathers all CEECs and former satellites of the USSR, except for the Czech Republic, which is clustered in the first model, and Bulgaria and Poland, which are found in the third model. Apart from the CEECs, we also find two further Mediterranean countries, Greece and Malta. This group of countries is below the mean for the twenty-eight in GDP per capita and levels of income and, apart from Malta and Romania, all of them have higher unemployment rates than the average for the twenty-eight. The Corruption Perception Index scores of these countries are, on average 4.98 out of ten, two points below the mean for the twenty-eight (Transparency International 2011). Regarding Inglehart's World Values Survey, all former USSR countries have 'survival values'. This means that these countries prioritize economic and physical security over self-expression values, which are linked to post-industrial societies that rely on effective democracies. Half these countries are not OECD member states and those within this model that are members of the OECD (Estonia, Greece, Hungary, and Slovakia) report between one and two points below the average in quality of life and material living conditions.

These countries are characterized by having a traditional approach to dealing with addictions, an issue tackled through a security-oriented perspective. In these countries, either the prime minister retains this responsibility or it is in hands of the ministries of the Interior, Justice, or Social Affairs, with the exception of Greece, where the Ministry of Health and Social Solidarity is in charge. Their focus is on supply reduction, prevention, and treatment, with only residual harm-reduction measures (see Box 7.1).

Taking into account alcohol consumption patterns, most of these countries have been classified as Central Eastern and Eastern European states. This

Box 7.1: Key elements of the traditional approach

- Countries embrace an individualistic and security-based approach, combined with a substance-based structure.
- These countries are European entrance points or routes in the trade of illicit substances.
- Policies are oriented towards reducing the supply of illicit drugs.
- The Ministry of the Interior is in charge of policy coordination. Countries tend to centralize policy-making and implementation.
- EU member states during the first decade of the 2000s (except for Greece and Malta).

means that these countries report higher rates of unrecorded consumption and are characterized by patterns of irregular heavy drinking (Popova et al. 2007; Zatonski et al. 2008). Spirits have played a 'relatively large role in most of these countries' (Anderson et al. 2012: 11), and differences between record-ed and unrecorded alcohol consumption are the highest of the twenty-eight countries.

According to the WHO (2013), the CEECs within this model are those with highest levels of alcohol-attributable 'standardized death rates' per 100,000 peo-ple. Rehm (2012: 5) states that 'the proportion of alcohol-attributable deaths in Central-eastern and Eastern Europe is much higher than in the southern region of the EU, for men more than twice as high'. More specifically, the author notes three explanations: a higher volume of drinking, an irregular pattern of drink-ing with high variation, and lower economic wealth. Hence, although these countries do not report the highest levels of recorded alcohol consumption, their patterns have an impact on the health of their population. To this, we should add a complementary fact, which is that surrogate and unrecorded alco-hol is widely consumed in CEECs (Lachenmeier et al. 2007). Greece and Malta, despite being clustered in this model, do not have the same patterns of alcohol consumption; neither do they report the high levels of alcohol-attributable standardized death rate.

The Baltic states (Estonia, Latvia, and Lithuania) can be differentiated from the rest of the countries in this model. All three have evidence-based regula-tions on alcohol and are the only states to have decriminalized possession of cannabis. Because of the alcohol-related problems of these countries, and in order to become harmonized with the EU trends, during the last few years

Central-Eastern European countries have become stricter and raised their excise duty on alcohol (Karlsson et al. 2012). In this respect, four CEEC within this model have stricter regulations on alcohol than the EU mean. Tobacco, on the other hand, is still loosely regulated and only Malta scores above the mid-point on the tobacco-control scale (Joossens and Raw 2010). We find in this cluster one of the highest percentages of tobacco smokers of the sample (see Fig. 5.2), except for Greece, Malta, and Slovakia.

The results show that these countries are mainly reactive and do not promote innovative policies. In this respect, none of them has top-rated best practices according to the EMCDDA, nor do they have injection rooms. We see higher levels of coincidence in the structure variables in this cluster than in the rest. In this sense, only Hungary is grouped separately, mainly because it involves non-profit organizations in the decision-making process. The cross-cutting commonalities in this domain are the presence of ad hoc coordinator bodies and the non-involvement of non-profit and private organizations in decision-making and implementation processes. Finally, the countries in this model present centralized patterns for policy-making and implementation. This is a key characteristic that, outside this model, is only shared by Cyprus and Luxembourg, the smallest countries in the model.

7.2 **Slovakia**

In Slovakia, the governance of addictions still is in an embryonic state. Slovakia focuses its attention on reducing supply without emphasizing harm-reduction measures, public health, or well-being. This country could therefore be regarded as an extreme example, since most of the countries in the traditional model have to some extent begun to cope with illicit substances. When it comes to dealing with drugs, the cornerstone of Slovakian policy is repression. As stated in the Slovakian National Anti-Drug Strategy for the period 2009–2012, promoting this policy does 'not mean the abandonment of the repressive part of the anti-drug policy, thus, reducing demand availability remains one of the basic strategies of preventing damage' (Government of the Slovak Republic 2009). Slovakia is, then, one of the very few countries that includes supply reduction in its top two policy priorities, which is interpreted as having a safety and disease approach. More specifically, the key objectives of the Slovakian strategy are:

1 To reduce the level of drug use in society and related risks and damage.

2 To reduce the supply of drugs with an emphasis on sanctioning the organized crime groups involved in illicit drug trafficking.

3 Enforcement of adherence to the law in connection with the production and distribution of drugs.

In Slovakia responsibility for the coordination and management of the governance of drugs and addictions lies with the Prime Minister (see Annex 29), although the ministries of Health and the Interior are in charge of demand and supply reduction, respectively. Second, although the law classifies substances according to the different effects they can produce on health, the penalties are not linked to this classification. Third, possession of illicit substances, even for personal use, is a criminal offence that carries the risk of a jail sentence.

Slovakia passed the first law intended to tackle illicit substances in 1967, when it was still part of Czechoslovakia. Two years after becoming an independent state, and in the transition period to access membership of the EU, the government passed the first Slovakian national strategy on drugs: the National Programme for the Fight against Drugs 1995–1998. This strategy was very much aligned with the European Drug Plan (1994–1999). As a candidate, Slovakia had to embrace EU recommendations in many fields, one of which was drug and addiction policies. However, in contrast to the Czech Republic, Slovakia opted for a safety and disease strategy, criminalizing drug possession and use, and focusing on public security rather than on health policies.

This effort to be aligned with EU values and perspectives is present in the 2009–2012 national strategy, which emphasizes scientific evidence, previous experience, pragmatic approaches, prevention, and individual as well as collective harm reduction. However, in practical terms, few of these practices aimed at dealing with illicit substances are implemented effectively.

Drug-related penalties are not linked to types of substance. However, since the approval of a new criminal code in 2006, Slovakia has become more aligned with the EU approach and has focused on punishing drug dealers, traffickers, and those who help legalize the profits of criminal drug activities (money laundering). The emphasis is now on supply containment and penalizing traffic and substance distribution instead of consumption of illicit substances. In fact, Slovakian penalties for possessing drugs are lower than the EU recommendations (Council of the EU 2004b).

Slovakia prioritizes prevention and treatment measures over harm-reduction actions. It is notably one of the EU countries with the fewest harm-reduction policies. Until 2010 there was no kind of provision of needle exchange programmes in prisons, nor substitution treatments for opiate dependents (Rhodes and Hedrich 2010).

One of the main features of Slovakian alcohol policies is its zero tolerance, which means that any BAC above 0.0 can be sanctioned. Nonetheless, and in contrast to the general EU trend, sanctions are administrative rather than penal. Despite this zero-tolerance policy, Slovakia does not require any licence for producing and commercializing beer and wine. Hence, some inconsistencies in the alcohol regulation are found, which makes Slovakia rate below the mean for the twenty-eight on the alcohol-policy scale.

Slovakian tobacco policies also rank low when compared to the twenty-eight and, as reported by Joossens and Raw (2010), there has been little activity to implement evidence-based regulations in this field. However, the most remarkable characteristic of Slovakia's policy is that it will be the last EU country to ratify the WHO Framework Convention for Tobacco Control in May 2014.

Despite not involving decentralized structures or other stakeholders in the decision-making process, selective and indicated prevention and treatment policies in Slovakia are implemented and delivered by non-profit organizations and private centres. Thus, policies are monitored centrally but implementation is delivered in collaboration with key stakeholders. Like every country in this model, Slovakia has an ad hoc body that coordinates drug and addiction policies: the permanent inter-ministerial Board of Ministers for Drug Addictions and Drug Control. This board is the responsibility of the Anti-drug Strategy Coordination Department, part of the foreign cooperation section of the Slovakian government. This is an interesting point, since Slovakia is the only country that links this coordination body with the Ministry of Foreign Affairs, which clearly denotes a will to promote cooperation with its neighbours to combat the traffic of illicit substances.

In summary, although Slovakia has theoretically embraced the EU guidelines, it still has not developed the necessary tools to implement these measures. It is worth remembering that, like most of the countries within this model, Slovakia became a member of the EU in 2004, just eleven years after attaining its independence.

7.3 **Estonia**

In Estonia, the Ministry of Social Affairs is in charge of the governance of addictions, working with the National Institute of Health Development, the Ministry of Justice, the Ministry of Internal Affairs, and the Ministry of Finance (see Annex 12). All of these are involved in the performance of the National Strategy for Prevention of Drug Addiction 2004–2012 (updated in 2009), which came into force in 2005 and replaced the former Alcohol and Drug Abuse Strategy of 1997.

The action plan has the following pillars: prevention, harm reduction, drug treatment and rehabilitation, reduction of supply, monitoring and evaluation, and drugs in prison. In 2011 Estonia had the highest rate of drug-related deaths in the EU. As noted by Estonian Public Broadcasting (2011), while 'on average, 21 people per million died in EU countries in the last two years; in Estonia it was 146 people per million'. One explanatory factor is that Estonia has one of the highest levels of heroin consumption in the EU. While the percentage of adult drug users taking heroin does not reach 1 per cent in the EU member states, in Estonia 1.52 per cent of adult drug users take heroin, making this country the EU member state with the highest level of opiate consumption (Lithuania Tribune 2010). Moreover, according to the UNODC World Drugs Report (UNODC 2011b: 30), 'the prevalence of HIV among injecting drug users in Estonia has reached 72 per cent'. These high levels of heroin consumption explain why harm reduction is one of the top priorities in the Estonian action plan. In 2003 the government started funding syringe exchange, and since then the number of NGOs aimed at reducing drug-related harm has increased significantly.

The national strategy includes alcohol and embraces a comprehensive policy that is shared only by Greece and Hungary among the countries of the traditional model. Estonia has developed strict regulation on alcohol and rates above the EU mean (Karlsson et al. 2012). Despite a policy trend oriented at restricting and reducing alcohol consumption, Estonia still has 195 places that sell alcohol per 100,000 citizens, compared to 4.5 places in Norway and Sweden (Joost 2010). Estonia's location also has consequences for its alcohol policies. The Estonian market is affected by the fact that Russian excise rates are one-third of those of Estonia. This, together with the fact that one of the most populated cities in Estonia (Narva) is on the border with Russia and that 80 per cent of the population of Narva are ethnic Russians, enhances the illicit cross-border trade of alcohol beverages (Elder 2008).

The Estonian ad hoc coordination body in the field of drugs and addictions is the Government Committee on Drug Prevention, which was established in 2006. Its main tasks are to revise the national drugs strategy, and update it if needed; draft the action plans for the implementation of the strategy; review annual reports; evaluate the implementation of the drug strategy; and draft an implementation report of the drug strategy for the government. The National Institute for Health Development is responsible for the implementation of treatment policies.

In summary, among the countries in the fourth model, Estonia appears to be moving easily towards a 'well-being and relational management' strategy and to be becoming more aligned with its Nordic neighbours (Finland, Sweden, and Norway).

7.4 **Greece**

Like its Mediterranean counterparts, Greece is facing one of the worst econom-ic crises the country has ever known. Bailed out by the troika in 2010, Greece is adjusting the public budget and implementing many austerity policies that have, so far, increased the unemployment rate and proved unable to boost its economy. According to the CIA (2012), because of its geostrategic location Greece is, like Bulgaria, a heroin gateway to the EU (see Annex 16). In this respect, Greece lies on the so-called Balkan route, which introduces heroin and cannabis coming from Central and South-East Asia to Central and Western Europe. This could explain Greece's repressive policies and safety and disease strategy.

The first Greek strategy on drugs and addictions was approved in 2006 and had the following pillars: coordination, demand reduction, supply reduction, international cooperation, training, research, and evaluation. Apart from train-ing, these are the same as those of the EU strategy (2005–2012). However, the focus of Greek policy is on improving access to treatment and minimizing wait-ing lists for substitution treatment. The main strategic sub-priorities are pre-vention and the fight against organized crime (Greece—EMCDDA, UMHRI, and REITOX National Report 2010). This focus can be seen in the budget allo-cation for treatment and prevention, €111m out of €155m, that is, 71.5 per cent of the total drugs and addictions policy budget (Greece—EMCDDA Country Overview 2011).

Although Greece does not decriminalize possession of illicit substances, the 1729/87 law of 1987 considers addicts to be patients rather than criminals, and states that when imposing sanctions and penalties it must be taken into account whether or not individuals are addicted to any substance. In 1995 an amend-ment of law 'placed particular emphasis on therapy, introducing the postpone-ment of the penal prosecution for drug law offenders that have undertaken therapeutic programmes'. Penalties for non-addicts can outweigh the EU rec-ommendations by five years (Council of the EU 2004b).

The Greek Ministry of Health and Social Solidarity is in charge of developing drug and addiction policies. This ministry also controls the principal body coordinating policies in this field: OKANA (Organization Against Drugs). Since 1995, OKANA 'plans, promotes, coordinates and implements the nation-al policy on prevention, treatment and rehabilitation of drug addictions, addresses the drug problem at national level, provide valid and documented information, raise public awareness and establishes and manages prevention centres, treatment units and social and professional reintegration centres' (OKANA 2012).

In order to deliver these services, OKANA collaborates with different treatment agencies, such as the Therapy Centre for Dependent Individuals (KETHEA) and the Rehabilitation Unit for Alcoholic Addicts (18ANO) as well as with local institutions, universities, the Greek Documentation and Information Centre on Drugs (EKTEPN), and the University Mental Health Research Institute (UMHRI). Despite being focused on universal prevention, Greece is increasing the number of selective and indicated interventions (Greece—EMCDDA, UMHRI and REITOX National Report 2010).

Greece reports levels below the EU average for three of the four substances; the exception is tobacco, which is slightly above the mid-point of the tobacco-control scale. Greece has similar patterns of alcohol consumption to those reported by Mediterranean countries. Legislation dating from 2002 puts the sale of alcohol on the same level as all goods, except for spirits (Karachaliou et al. 2005). There is no specific law on sales of alcohol (Amphora 2012).

The economic crisis has had pernicious effects on drug use in Greece, increasing the consumption level of some substances. Specifically, it has had an effect on heroin consumption, especially among injecting drug users who do not have access to needle exchange and have greater difficulty in receiving proper substitution treatments, with an increase of drug-related cases of HIV (European Coalition for Just and Effective Drug Policies 2012). As noted in the same report, the rise of unemployment combined with the budgetary cuts in Greece may have significant negative effects on the population.

7.5 **Hungary**

Like the majority of the countries in this model, Hungary's policy on drugs and addictions has been progressively converging with general EU trends since the country regained its independence in 1990. Hungarian levels of income and GDP per capita are similar to those of the Baltic countries (see Annex 17).

The objectives of Hungarian drugs and addiction polices are to 'improve the health status of the society, to increase social safety, and to reduce the rate of drug consumption, the harms, risks, and damages of the use of legal and illicit drugs' (Hungary—-EMCDDA National Drug Strategy 2012). To accomplish these objectives, the national strategy tackles drug-related issues through three pillars: prevention and community intervention; treatment, care, and harm reduction; and supply reduction.

The Ministry of Social Affairs and Labour is in charge of coordinating drugs and addictions policy and also leads the Coordination Committee on Drug Affairs, the ad hoc body in charge of coordinating drug policies across Hungary. The safety and disease approach embraced by Hungary can be seen in its drug-related expenditure, which, in 2007, was mainly aimed at enhancing law enforcement (66 per cent of total expenditure), while treatment and harm reduction together did not exceed 15 per cent of the total budget (EMCDDA 2013a). Moreover, Hungarian law imposes life imprisonment for drug-related offences, a strict policy that is not contemplated in the EU recommendations.

Penalties are not linked to drug type, so cannabis consumption is considered a major offence and incurs penal consequences similar to those imposed for heroin consumption. One possible explanation of this restrictive vision is that Hungary has traditionally been a transit country for heroin trafficked along the Balkan route to Western Europe. However, it is worth noting that in 2003 the Hungarian government amended the criminal code, reducing the maximum sentence if the offender is an addict and removing 'consumption' as a specific offence.

Although Hungary reports one of the strictest BAC levels among the sample (it implements zero tolerance), it still ranks as one of the lowest countries in the cluster on the alcohol-policy scale. The low score on the tobacco-control scale can be considered a key explanatory factor for the 38 per cent of smokers in this country, the highest percentage among the twenty-eight and well above the mean (29 per cent). As Joossens and Raw (2010) note, Hungary has a powerful tobacco industry, which makes it difficult to approve evidence-based regulations.

Hungary tackles licit and illicit substances together. The Hungarian Coordination Committee on Drug Affairs includes representatives from all ministries and national institutions concerned as well as representatives from four different non-profit organizations. It is the only country in the model that involves non-profit organizations (which provide treatment at regional level) in the decision-making process.

7.6 Latvia

The Ministry of the Interior is in charge of governing addictions in Latvia (see Annex 20), although the Ministry of Health has significant input. Drug treatment is mainly delivered by institutions that operate under the supervision of the Ministry of Health and are funded by the National Health Service budget. In 1993 the National Drug policy established the following principles to cope with drug-related problems and addictions:

1 To reduce drug availability.

2 To control use of legal substances.

3 To ensure primary and secondary prevention programmes.

4 To facilitate the treatment of addicts.

Since then, the approach of Latvia's ad hoc coordination body (the Drug Control and Drug Addiction Restriction Coordination Council) has adapted to take into account international guidelines, and has introduced new concepts and policies, such as harm reduction. The main objectives of the 2011–2017 strategy are to reduce acceptance of illicit drug use, and the harm caused by it; to enhance the accessibility and effectiveness of healthcare services provided to drug users; and to reduce the availability of illicit drugs. One of the goals is to reduce the harm caused to society, rather than to the drug user. This is reinforced by the fact that Latvia, Estonia, and Lithuania are the only countries in this model that decriminalize drug possession.

While Latvia's strategy, like that of its Baltic counterparts, can be distinguished from that of the other countries in this model—mainly because it decriminalizes possession of illicit substances and has more harm-reduction policies—its structure is very similar. Latvia has an ad hoc coordinator body and involves more than 50 per cent of its ministries in the governance of addictions; however, it does not devolve policy-making and implementation to decentralized structures.

Latvia's main drug problem is its high level of heroin trafficking—the three Baltic countries are on the so-called Silk Route, which brings Afghan heroin through the central Asian states and Russia—and consumption. To tackle these, Latvia developed the National Programme for Limiting HIV and AIDS 2009–2013. Two major harm-reduction responses are carried out in Latvia: opiate substitution programmes and a network of low-threshold centres (LTCs) for injecting drug users. LTCs provide a wide range of low-threshold services: needle exchange, outreach, voluntary HIV counselling and testing, HCV testing, disinfectants, condoms, group and individual risk-reduction information, education, etc.

Latvia's approach to alcohol is focused on regulating production and sales. A licence is required to produce and sell alcoholic products, and there are restrictions regarding the places and the hours in which alcohol can be sold. The BAC level for driving must be 0.05 per cent or less, a low percentage that is aligned with the regulative approach of the country. In summary, Latvia rates above the EU mean on the alcohol-policy scale. The main alcohol problem in the country is illicit trade. According to the Alcohol Producers and Traders Association, illicit trade of alcohol represents between 35 and 40 per cent of the total Latvian market (Baltic News Network 2012). Notwithstanding, the anti-alcohol advocacy organization, Sobriety Union, has asked the government to embrace Scandinavian policies of restricting takeaway alcohol sales to governmental monopolies and banning the advertising of alcohol (Joost 2010). Like every country in this model, Latvia ranks below the mid-point on the tobacco-control scale, although the percentage of smokers in the country outweighs the mean for the twenty-eight. Finally, although non-profit organizations are not involved in decision-making, the national government established agreements with four institutions (three Christian and one NGO) to provide rehabilitation programmes.

7.7 Lithuania

Lithuania passed its first national strategy in 2010, the National Programme on Drug Control and Prevention of Drug Addiction 2010–2016, which prioritizes prevention of consumption, especially among young people. The national strategy prioritizes four areas: demand reduction, among children and youth in particular; supply reduction; cooperation and coordination; IT and scientific research.

Like its Baltic neighbours, Lithuania is a remarkable case because it is among the few countries within this model that decriminalize the possession of illicit substances and ranks above the mean of the twenty-eight on the alcohol-policy scale (see Annex 21). Moreover, Lithuania is one of the few countries to introduce a public-health concept in its national strategy. Lithuania does not have a Ministry of Health in charge of addiction policies. Instead, the institution in charge of drug and addiction policies is the government's Drug Control Department, which carries out monitoring and analysis of communications on the topic of psychoactive substance use throughout the country. Interestingly, the coordination, implementation, and provision of drug treatment is conducted at the local level. Drug treatment is provided by national or local public institutions, jointly with private and non-profit organizations. Supply reduction is still one of the main priorities of the national strategy jointly with the reduction of the illicit use of addictive substances.

Lithuania has some internationally recognized policies in this field, such as 'Training for professionals', which aims to build and maintain contact with members of the municipal drug control commission (EMCDDA 2011c). Universal prevention, one of the main targets of the national strategy, is mainly implemented by the Ministry of Education and Sciences, which delivers prevention for legal and illicit substances.

Since 1997 the Vilnius Centre for Dependence Diseases in collaboration with the Open Society Foundation in Lithuania—both private centres—have been implementing low-threshold programmes for injecting drug users. In 2006, almost ten years later, the Ministry of Health provided the minimum criteria to implement these services. The main focus, however, is on information and counselling; harm-reduction policies are mainly implemented by public institutions and businesses. However, research in 2008 showed high intolerance on the part of pharmacy personnel towards injecting drug users, and since then no targeted programme for harm reduction has considered pharmacies as potential partners (Lithuania—EMCDDA Country Overview 2011).

In summary, the structure of this country is very similar to that of the other countries within this model. However, it is the only country to include the term 'addiction' in its national strategy and to take a comprehensive view that goes beyond what happens with each substance and tries to respond to the overall problem.

7.8 **Malta**

Malta is a special case due to its small size; it represents 0.01 per cent of the territory of the twenty-eight countries and 0.08 per cent of the overall population. Maltese levels of alcohol, tobacco, and cannabis consumption are significantly below the EU average; however, it has higher heroin prevalence levels than the EU average (see Annex 23). The main objectives of the Maltese national strategy, passed in 2008, are:

1 Ensuring a high level of security to the general public and a high level of health protection.

2 Well-being.

3 Social cohesion.

Malta and Bulgaria are the only EU member states to introduce well-being as an objective of their strategy. The Maltese strategy is focused on improving the quality of drug users' services and the main points are very similar to the EU strategy: coordination; legal and judicial framework; supply reduction; demand reduction; monitoring and international cooperation.

The Ministry of Justice, Dialogue and the Family is responsible for addiction policies. It aims to 'promote the development of a secure, just, and inclusive society where every citizen's rights and freedoms are safeguarded in an equitable and secure environment' (Government of Malta 2012). The safety and disease strategy of the Maltese government is reaffirmed by the fact that the trafficking of cannabis or cocaine is punishable with similar sentencing; drug classification does not determine penalties. The main agency implementing preventive and treatment policies is the National Agency on Drugs, known as Sedqa. On the non-profit side, we find Caritas and the OASI Foundation, which are partially funded by local governments and are focused on treatment.

As noted, Malta is one of the few countries including well-being and public health among its aims. Theoretically, this should mean that this country has a well-being and relational approach strategy; however, apart from these two characteristics, Malta rates above the mid-point on the tobacco-control scale and on supply reduction, which is not a top priority in the national strategy.

The Maltese strategy deals with illicit drugs and alcohol, with the focus on illicit drugs and the abuse of medication. Most of the actions established in the strategy are intended to reduce the demand for drugs among Maltese citizens. Under the responsibility of the Ministry of Social Policies, the National Coordinating Unit for Drugs and Alcohol prepares policy documents and amendments.

Malta reports the lowest level of alcohol consumption in the EU (Joossens and Raw 2010; see Fig. 5.4), despite defining alcoholic beverages as those containing 2 per cent of alcohol concentration (above the EU average). Furthermore, it has one of the highest BAC levels for drinking and driving, has no restrictive measures on alcohol advertising, and does not implement random alcohol tests. The *Times of Malta* reported that, according to an EU-wide survey, 73 per cent of Maltese citizens want the levels of BAC to be lowered for young and novice drivers (Camilleri 2010).

7.9 **Romania**

Romania is the largest country in this cluster and has the largest population (see Annex 28). The second national strategy of the Romanian government, which covers 2005–2012, aims to 'develop an integrated system of institutional and public services to ensure the reduction of drug use, adequate medical, psychological and social assistance for drug users, and streamlined activities for preventing and countering the trafficking and production of illicit drugs and precursors' (Romania—EMCDDA Country Overview 2011). Following the model of the EU strategy, and like many countries within this model, Romania bases its strategy on demand reduction, supply reduction, international cooperation, information and evaluation, and inter-agency coordination.

The Romanian strategy is clearly aligned with a safety and disease approach. Romania has a long trajectory legislating illicit substances—its first law dates back to 1928. After Bulgaria and Greece, Romania is one of the EU countries most affected by the Balkan Route, and supply reduction is a high-priority issue for the Romanian authorities (Government of Romania 2005). Although drug consumption has been decriminalized per se, drug possession is still a criminal offence.

Apart from this, Romania's primary policies for prevention are mainly universal and delivered through schools. While selective prevention is mostly targeted at Roma groups, the prison population, former drug users, victims of family violence, and young adults leaving care, indicated prevention interventions remain isolated and rare. Harm-reduction measures are not as developed as prevention and treatment measures. Moreover, until 2010, prevention activities targeting drug-related infectious diseases related to injection were mainly financed under the Global Fund to Fight AIDS, Tuberculosis and Malaria, and were implemented by NGOs. Interestingly, most syringe programmes and harm-reduction services are funded by international organizations: either the UN or the EU.

Romania ranks above the EU mean on the alcohol-policy scale. The government requires licences for the production, retail sale, and distribution of alcoholic beverages among other evidence-based regulative measures. Although it rates below the mid-point of the tobacco-control scale, it is getting closer to this point (Joossens and Raw 2010). Since its entrance into the EU, Romania has increased the duty on tobacco.

Since 2002, the National Anti-drug Agency (NAA), under the Ministry of the Interior and Administrative Reform, has coordinated the governance of addictions. Prevention campaigns are organized by the NAA jointly with the Ministry of Education, Innovation and Research together with non-governmental representatives from NGOs and schools. The NAA has set up a network of forty-seven drug-prevention, evaluation, and counselling centres through which the agency coordinates the implementation of drug-related policies. Furthermore, treatment policies are delivered by public, private, and non-profit organizations.

7.10 **Conclusion to Model 4 in Europe**

In this model we primarily find Central and Eastern European countries that became EU member states during the first decade of the twenty-first century. The exceptions are Greece and Malta, which are Mediterranean countries in the welfare state regimes classification (Ferrera 1996). As former satellites of the USSR, most of these countries have not been classified in any of the welfare state regimes taken into account. While the first model has been classified as having a well-being and relational management approach, combined with a comprehensive structure, countries within this model are characterized by the opposite trends in both domains. Hence, countries in the traditional model have aggregated characteristics that cluster them into a safety and disease strategy, combined with a substance-based approach.

More specifically, most of the countries give the responsibility for managing drug and addiction policies to the prime minister, the Ministry of the Interior, the Ministry of Justice, or the Ministry of Social Affairs. Moreover none of them determines penalties according to drug classification. Since regaining their independence from the USSR, these countries have been making an effort to align their governance of addictions with that promoted by the EU. Most have similarly structured national strategies with almost the same chapters as those in the EU strategies. Nevertheless, in practical terms, they continue to criminalize drug use and possession and their broad approach is more safety- and disease-oriented than that promoted by the EU.

We found very little involvement of public, private, and non-profit stakeholders in the decision-making process and regional administrations are involved neither in policy-making nor in the implementation process.

Finally, in this group the Baltic countries seem to be approaching a more well-being and relational strategy by decriminalizing possession of illicit substances and implementing strict and evidence-based regulation of alcohol. We believe that proximity with the Nordic countries and membership of the Nordic alcohol and drug policy (NordAN) has influenced the policies of the Baltic countries, especially towards alcohol.

Chapter 8

Conclusion: The key to understanding the governance of addictions in Europe

8.1 European government policies on addictions: A comparative analysis

This book presents comparative, multi-disciplinary research (including public management, health, political science, sociology, economics, and law) that develops an explanatory framework for understanding how governments formulate and implement addiction policies in Europe. Through an in-depth analysis of the twenty-seven EU member states, plus Norway, we present four European models of governance of addictions. For this purpose, four substances are taken into account—heroin, cannabis, alcohol, and tobacco.

The study focuses on policies and governance practices from the beginning of 2005 to the end of 2011. Nonetheless, to provide a historical perspective and see the evolution of governance, documents from 1980 to 2012 have been taken into account. The methodology is mainly qualitative, although supported by large quantitative databases. We gathered information from national strategies and action plans, documents on specific substances and penalties imposed, national reports and documents produced by international organizations and agencies (the WHO, the UN, and the European Monitoring Centre for Drugs and Drug Addictions). To complement this official information, eighteen interviews with experts from fourteen EU countries were conducted, and we followed up media coverage.

Which are the current public policies to deal with addictions in Europe? The main aim of our research has been to answer this question. To this end, we have devised an interpretative key that has enabled us to analyse the various models for action employed by European governments and identify the basic elements to analyse and understand public policies action on governance of addictions. We have created a frame to understand and compare the various models used by European governments (see Fig. 8.1). With it we identify four European models: (1) the trend-setters in illicit substances model; (2) the regulation of legal substances model; (3) the transitioning model; and (4) the traditional

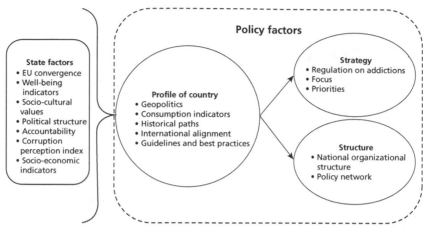

Fig. 8.1 The governance of addictions in Europe

model. This in turn permits an analysis of the governance of addictions in Europe: (a) government strategies and policies on addictions; (b) decision-making processes and organizational structures developed; (c) the new links between actors to generate a policy shift on the governance of addictions.

8.2 **Governance framework and trends**

By taking governance as our reference framework, instead of government, we assume that, as with many other public issues, addictions can no longer be tackled by governments alone. There is a need to produce better results through collaboration and to promote the involvement of various organizations in order to maximize the outcomes to society and social well-being. Research institutions, non-profit organizations, addicts, families, professionals, and even businesses are already part not only of a pluralist provision of services (co-production), but also of a pluralist process for policy design and implementation. There are three key provisos to this approach:

1 The leading role in determining the strategy of the public policy for addictions should always be in public sector hands to enhance societal well-being.

2 An evolved co-production system has to find ways of avoiding co-optation by both industry and NGOs dependent on public budgets.

3 Transparency, checks, and balances should be ensured as the drivers to increase evidence-based impact in decision-making.

Chapter 1 introduces three trends in the current governance of addictions: decriminalization of the use and possession of illicit substances, broader acceptance of harm-reduction perspectives, and an increased focus on policy scales based on evidence-based regulations for legal substances. This is an ongoing contested issue between scientists and public officials. Evidence-based policies are without doubt the most effective way to deal with addictions, but public management may not systematically translate them fully into public action. In democracies, public policies are social constructs designed to deal with social problems, the fruit of dialogue between principles, ideologies, past history, collective action, scope, and costs, among others. To avoid confrontation between two desirable goals (democracy and evidence-based approaches), policy windows of opportunity should be sought by evidence-bearers, to align policy cycles and best responses to social needs.

The major impacts of these trends are presented in the first and the second models. The first, the trend-setters in illicit substances model, gathers a group of countries that have passed laws to decriminalize the use and possession of illicit substances and, at the same time, give significant importance to harm-reduction policies, a growing practice in these countries. Countries in the second model, regulation of legal substances, do not focus on decriminalization, but implement evidence-based regulations aimed at reducing the levels of alcohol and tobacco consumption, and enhancing societal well-being. The other two models, transitioning and traditional, are only starting to include some of these trends.

None of the models described in this book embraces these three trends simultaneously, showing that policy-making is subject to contingency factors, such as path-dependency frames, as well as to different forces and traditions that cannot be ignored when reframing previous approaches. We should ask whether these trends are mutually incompatible. Theoretically this should not be the case; however, reality proves very different. Those countries embracing a regulatory approach do not have many decriminalization and harm-reduction policies—and vice versa.

A consolidated tendency towards a health approach is shown by placing the major responsibility for the governance of drugs and addiction under the Ministry of Health. And although the terms 'public health' and 'well-being' are not used in official documents, our measures show that these are the outcomes countries are pursuing. Conversely, the two countries that do use this wording in their national strategies consider them more as a future reference point for addictions than a real implementation. Another trend revealed by the results is that most countries put prevention, demand reduction, or harm reduction high among their priorities, while supply reduction is losing impetus, at least in national strategies. Injection rooms have not yet become part of an extended programme in Europe, and we find them only in the first model. The results also show stricter alcohol policies in countries where spirits are consumed than in beer- and wine-producing countries. Finally, almost all countries have best practices (although only eight reach the EMCDDA's more demanding level 3), but few are internationally known.

Although there is a tendency to aggregate illicit substances and alcohol, there is still a lack of comprehensive strategies that include all substances and behaviours that generate problems related to heavy use. The countries approaching a more comprehensive approach are those that focus on harm reduction and decriminalization of drug consumption, and have a public-health orientation. The number of ministries involved in the national strategy, as a proxy to a holistic structural approach to the issue, does not indicate a tendency in Europe. It is true that more ministries are involved than traditionally (especially Health, the Interior, Justice, and the office of the prime minister), but the composition of cabinets is so contingent to individual countries that the aggregation of responsibilities in each country makes it difficult to infer any consequences. Finally, there is a common trend in all countries in the sample: all of them have created an ad hoc body to coordinate the public policy for addictions among governments and stakeholders.

As presented in Figs 2.1 and 2.2, most national policies for addictions and action plans are still split into two groups, legal and illicit substances, with the latter split further into demand and supply reduction. Despite eager efforts among the scientific community to find innovative approaches to cross-cutting policy-making, the reality is that this division is very present across Europe.

Regarding stakeholder participation, while differences arise between member states, mainly due to their historical, cultural, and political backgrounds, we can identify a cross-country pattern across Europe embedding the following characteristics:

1 A decision-making process led by the government, in collaboration with stakeholders—from NGOs to businesses.

2 Implementation mainly carried out by non-profit organizations and secondarily by the government—here the role of businesses is controversial and implementation is normally carried out by their foundations. The involvement of non-profit organizations, and to a lesser extent foundations, can be seen particularly in policies oriented towards reducing the demand for illicit substances (treatment, prevention, harm reduction, and social reintegration).

3 An evaluation of the policies conducted by governments in collaboration with research institutes and non-profit organizations.

In contrast to the EU, member states do not tend to have participatory platforms incorporating the three sectors (government, businesses and NGOs).

The main difference between the EU and the models of its member states is that the former does not have the capacity to implement policies, which is retained by each member state. The most relevant role for the EU is decision-making, which is carried out through participatory platforms, multi-stakeholder forums, and public consultations aimed at receiving inputs, comments, amendments, and observations from relevant stakeholders in the field of addictions. The roles of the European Civil Society Forum on Drugs (CSF) and the Alcohol and Health Forum are especially noteworthy. The CSF meets once a year and serves as a platform for informal exchanges of views and information between the Commission and civil society organizations (EC-DG Justice 2011). The Alcohol and Health Forum, on the other hand, gathers relevant stakeholders at EU level to compare approaches and actions to cope with alcohol-related harm (EC-DG Health 2011). In summary, the main roles of these multi-stakeholder platforms are to participate in EU public consultations and make their voices heard and their interests more visible to public institutions.

Furthermore, both the third sector and businesses aim to influence EU decision-making processes directly, the former through a research-based approach and the latter through lobby pressures.

8.3 **Four models of governance of addictions in Europe**

In order to answer the question regarding addiction models in Europe we analyse the governance of addictions in the EU member states, plus Norway. Obviously every country has its own particularities and generalization is always difficult, even more when it comes to such a sensitive policy as addictions. However, this is a worthwhile effort and (to our knowledge) is the first attempt to cluster twenty-eight countries according to their public policies on addictions (comparing two legal and two illicit substances). For that we have conducted a bottom-up research process, departing from national information to group countries. The final classification is the result of qualitative and quantitative grand comparisons.

The models have been built on the basis of two constructs: strategy and structure (see Fig. 8.1). These constructs allowed us to analyse similarities and differences between countries and establish four models of governance of addictions in Europe (see Table 8.1).

Each model stresses a dominant perspective, although this does not exclude embracing other characteristics. The trend-setters in illicit substances model (model 1), is mainly characterized by its strategy towards illicit substances,

Table 8.1 Models of governance of addictions in Europe

Model	Characteristics	Countries
Trend-setters in illicit substances	Combine a well-being and relational management strategy with a comprehensive structure. Focus on illicit substances through harm reduction. Low rankers on legal policy scales.	Belgium, Czech Republic, Germany, Italy, Luxemburg, Netherlands, Portugal, and Spain
Regulation of legal substances	Combine a well-being and relational management strategy with a comprehensive structure. Focus on legal substances (tobacco and alcohol). No decriminalization of possession.	Finland, France, Ireland, Norway, Sweden, and the UK
Transitioning model	Countries transitioning, mostly from the traditional model to a more comprehensive one, but still with a substance separation approach. Do not decriminalize possession.	Austria, Bulgaria, Cyprus, Denmark, Poland, and Slovenia
Traditional approach	These countries embrace an individualistic and safety- and disease-based approach, combined with an organizational structure based on approaching substances separately.	Estonia, Greece, Hungary, Latvia, Lithuania, Malta, Romania, and Slovakia

which gives considerable importance to harm-reduction policies. Another distinctive characteristic of this model is the fact that the eight countries it comprises decriminalize possession of illicit substances. This is a socially controverted measure and it takes time for countries to get around to implementing it. Thus, countries in model 1 have normally undergone lengthy debate and sustained efforts in conjunction with key stakeholders to make decriminalization happen.

A second commonality of the countries in this model is their low ranking on the alcohol and tobacco scales. Model 1 introduces evidence-based policies to deal with illicit substances, shifting from a repressive to a more liberal approach. However, when it comes to the application of evidence-based scales for legal substances, states in the first model still do not fully include measures related to production, distribution, age limits, taxes, and advertising and marketing. Finally, most of the countries in model 1 have a long trajectory legislating drugs and addictions. Their governance of addictions is coordinated between most of the existing government ministries, and finally, those countries decentralize policy-making and implementation to multi-level governance structures (regional and/or local governments).

The countries in the regulation of legal substances model (model 2) have developed extensive evidence-based regulation for alcohol and tobacco, and their policies on legal substances are aligned with a well-being and relational management strategy. The countries in model 2 rank above the mean on both alcohol and tobacco scales, signifying that, unlike model 1, these countries aim to reduce the levels of consumption of legal substances, prevent heavy use over time, and improve the overall well-being of the population. Nevertheless, none of these six countries decriminalizes illicit substances.

These countries also have complex organizational structures to deal with addictions. Implementation is decentralized into multi-level organizational structures; non-profit organizations are involved in decision-making, and there is a sound trajectory for dealing with drugs. Therefore, countries in model 2 can be described as having a comprehensive structure that is combined, at least for legal substances, with a well-being and relational management approach. In order to boost this approach, countries within this model could extend it towards illicit substances.

The transitioning model (model 3), as its name implies, groups six countries that are moving towards one of the other three models. In general terms, this model is characterized by being closer to the safety and disease strategy than to the well-being and relational management approach. However, most of the countries in model 3 are shifting their policies and embracing well-being and relational management measures, such as best practices and evidence-based regulation for alcohol, which makes it safe to assume that sooner or later they will attain the characteristics of either model 1 or model 2. On the other hand, the organizational structure of these countries to deal with addictions policy is, in most of the cases, closer to a comprehensive than to a substance-based approach.

Finally, all the countries in the traditional model (model 4), except for Greece and Malta, became EU member states during the first decade of the twenty-first century. This means that, when interpreting results, we must take into account that most of these countries are still incorporating most of the guidelines and the well-being and relational management strategy promoted by the EU. They do not possess the necessary trajectory to develop the EU way of dealing with addictions. These countries' policies are more oriented towards reducing supply than to reducing demand for illicit drugs, and the Ministry of the Interior is normally in charge of drugs policy. They also tend to centralize policy-making and implementation. Broadly, these countries still have to develop a sound strategy and a comprehensive structure to cope with addictions. In this sense, they have been classified as having a safety and disease strategy combined with a substance-based structure.

Geopolitically, these countries are entrance points on the routes of illicit substances and alcohol and tobacco smuggling into Europe, which helps explain their supply reduction approach. However, it seems clear that countries in model 4 will have to find a balance between supply reduction and well-being approaches in the future to align with neighbouring countries.

The results from our research lead to the conclusion that strategy determines structure in the governance of addictions in Europe. Thus, when a country embraces a well-being and relational management strategy, it consequently develops a more comprehensive organizational structure. Hence, the more harm-reduction, regulation, and decriminalization policies a country has, the more involvement of multi-level governance and multi-stakeholder participation it needs. The finding that strategy determines structure is also justified by the fact that none of the twenty-eight countries analysed has a well-being and relational management strategy combined with a substance-based structure.

8.4 **The contingent comparative approach to addictions**

If we compare the final European models for the governance of addictions with former studies classifying countries in Europe, such as Esping-Andersen (1990), Ferrera (1996), Hall and Soskice (2001), Bohle and Greskovits (2006), Albareda et al. (2007), the GINI coefficient and other economic indicators (Eurostat 2011a, 2011b), the OECD Better Life Initiative variables (OECD 2011a), sustainable governance indicators (2011), Transparency International Corruption Perception Index (2011), and Inglehart's World Values Survey (2012), we conclude that there is no exact match between them and the governance of addictions. Neither have we found complete coincidence between studies related to consumption of a single substance, such as the one undertaken by Anderson et al. (2012) for alcohol patterns, and our final classification. The governance of addictions has its own levers, coming from the contingent combination of context (state factors) and the logistics of policy (strategy and structure).

For example, regarding the welfare state regime and the models of governance of addictions, model 1 gathers continental and Mediterranean countries; model 2 integrates Nordic, Anglo-Saxon, and continental countries; model 3 clusters continental, eastern, and Mediterranean countries; and model 4 consists of mainly Eastern European countries with two non-CEEC states. We cannot therefore state that the welfare state regimes determine public policies for addictions, although they are highly influenced by them. The same stands for the other classifications.

However, we can note some interesting contextual matches within the models. Firstly, all the CEECs in model 4 have survival rather than self-expression values, except for Greece. This means that their citizens put the emphasis on economic and physical security; they are ethno-centric and report low levels of trust and tolerance. Furthermore, as Anderson et al. (2012) present, there are notorious coincidences if we cross Esping-Andersen's work and the different patterns of alcohol consumption in Europe.

All countries in model 2 report above the average for the twenty-eight in economic indicators (Eurostat 2011a), and also in quality of life and material living conditions (OECD 2011b). This is mainly due to the presence of the Nordic countries, which rate among the top in most of the indicators. On the other side of the coin we find countries in model 4 that rate below the average for the twenty-eight in all contextual indicators. Model 1 shows that Mediterranean countries rate below the mean while continental countries have better rates. In model 3 there is more divergence between countries.

8.5 **Research limitations**

Our research has many limitations. In our research we devoted a huge effort towards obtaining comparable data in order to classify the different countries. It was a massive task to compile information on the twenty-eight countries, especially to find all the information needed, due to the lack of standardization of data, access to information, and the different languages involved.

The hardest element of this was to obtain the names of stakeholders participating in policy-making and information about budgets devoted to the provision of policies on addictions, which part of the policy cycle third parties participate in, or what capacity for manoeuvre they have. At the EU level it has been impossible to create a census with accurate information on the participation of the business or non-profit sectors.

Finally, because our focus has been at the national level, we have omitted in-depth information about decentralization and devolution processes from this book. They were, of course, taken into account when analysing each country, but our aim was to focus on strategies at the EU level, thus omitting this fine-grain approach. It will be important for future research to develop the same analysis at regional and local levels, particularly because policies on addictions are highly decentralized in Europe, at least in their implementation.

8.6 **Final remarks**

Addiction issues will always be there, and it is the responsibility of governments and societies to fight, as much as possible, their negative effects. Better governance of addictions, far from the widely known 'war against drugs', is possible. As our research shows, some countries have already made outstanding achievements in building complex solutions to complex problems. So far, none of the four models in Europe has been able to maximize results for both licit and illicit substances, while pursuing societal well-being. There is still room for improvement in all four models. The challenge now is how to take the best from the different models and combine this into one governance model when there are so many variables and stakeholders involved.

An EU-wide approach proves difficult, since historical paths, socio-economic standards, values, and geostrategic locations affect levels of consumption and ultimately the governance of addictions. Nonetheless, as the EU has shown in the last two decades, it is useful to establish minimum requirements and recommendations in order to promote harmonization, especially driven by evidence-based research. Through our analysis of the different countries, national strategies, and action plans, we can conclude that there is a clear tendency towards harmonization to make countries more aligned with the strategies and action plans passed at EU level. The EU promotes a comprehensive policy structure for addictions and lifestyles, while embracing a co-production strategy (relational management) for a well-being outcome. The analysis of the EU approach shows that it itself sits between the first and the second model in the upper-right quadrant.

A historical analysis of documents show that current country positions in these models are not fixed. They are highly dependent on ideological changes, socio-economic conditions, political leadership, and policy transfers. In 2013 we still saw countries changing models for addictions as a result of issues contested in elections. All countries depart from an individual approach to addictions (the far end of the safety and disease approach), with a compilation of drug control laws and mental health initiatives, and from there they develop different answers to addictions, at different speeds. Taking Fig. 8.2, we can anticipate the strong influence of the accession processes to the EU in the evolution of the different models, combined with a specific approach to legal and illicit substances. In Europe there is a tendency for models to move from the bottom-left quadrant, crossing the upper-left to the upper-right. The fact that none of the countries analysed has a well-being and relational strategy combined with a substance-based structure propels this.

Finally, in the years to come, we will have to take into account the effects of the economic crisis in Europe to measure how countries are impacted by the need to balance prolonged austerity measures with high-quality addictions policies, and in turn how this will impact the classification of the countries in the models. In some countries, high levels of debt have led to a reduction in

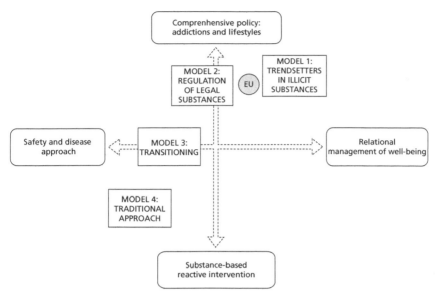

Fig. 8.2 Governance of addictions: European models and visions

social services budgets. Simultaneously, there is also the risk that substance use and abuse will increase as a consequence of high unemployment rates. However, some countries deeply affected by the crisis, such as Portugal, stand out for their innovative policies, demonstrating that these factors are not mutually exclusive. In this respect, Portugal is preparing a new national strategy that will go beyond the supply and demand division and deal with addictions through environments.

We have also seen some policy limitation in the research. The creation of forums and participatory platforms is not a guarantee of the real involvement of civil society and corporations in the policy-making and implementation processes. In future it will be necessary to assess the true extent to which cross-cutting approaches are necessary, useful, or implemented.

Globalization trends could also impact on future European policies on addictions. The traditional politics of international relations is starting to be questioned by developing countries, the main producers of illicit substances. As a result, there is increasing consensus across Latin American countries to open a debate on drugs policy and its effectiveness, questioning why they have to suffer the externalities of international agreements while the main consumers of illicit drugs are in developed countries. This conflicts with the USA's 'war against drugs', which opposes this debate. Meanwhile the EU seems unprepared to tackle this debate since it still lacks internal consensus among member states.

Annexes

Annex 1: Semi-structured interviews with experts and scientists

Introduction

This interview is part of ALICE RAP's research aimed at identifying and describing the typologies of governance of addictions (heroin, cannabis, tobacco, alcohol, but not gambling) across Europe.

Instructions

The interview is organized in three main parts. When possible, please provide short and concrete answers. It will be recorded. The interview proceeds as follows: first we will ask you questions about your expertise; then we will ask about key governance of addictions domains for your country. Finally we will ask how you see the international context and its influence on national policies.

About the interviewee

1 Could you briefly describe your current work position telling us the institution you belong to and your principal tasks?

2 Are you an expert on a specific substance? If so, which one?

3 On a 1–5 scale (1 is least and 5 most), please rate your level of expertise at national level on governance of addictions.

4 In a 1–5 scale (1 is least and 5 most), please rate your level of expertise at international level on governance of addictions.

National level

1 Do you think that the policy-making on addictions in your country is based on a national consensus that goes beyond who is governing the country?

2 How would you describe the relation between politicians, practitioners, and experts in the public policy on addictions?

3 Is it done by the government alone or with the collaboration of private and non-profit actors?

4 What is the role of industry in the policy-making process?

5 What are the main organizations involved in implementing policies on addictions in your country? Are they public, private, or non-profit organizations?

6 Could you briefly describe the role of the industry (alcohol and tobacco), its influence on the policy-making of addictions and in the implementation process?

7 Does the national strategy of your country include all substances? Why? Why not?

8. What would you say is the main focus of the current policy in your country?

9 Could you rank them from 1 to 8, 1 being the most important focus and 8 the least?

(1) Prevention

(2) Treatment

(3) Harm reduction

(4) Social assistance/reintegration programs

(5) Trade policies

(6) Production policies

(7) Cooperation (national or international)

(8) Research, monitoring

(9) Other

10 We would like to know what is the main factor affecting the governance of addictions. Could you rank the following from 1 to 6, where 1 is the most important factor and 6 the least?

(1) Levels of consumption

(2) International alignment

(3) Social pressure from drug addicts and their environment

(4) Social pressure from professionals in the field

(5) Pressure from the private sector

(6) Historical facts

(7) Other

11 In terms of addiction policy, can you identify a country like yours? Which and why?

12 If you could choose a country to resemble regarding the governance of addictions, which would it be and why?

13 If you were a policy-maker, what would you change in the current governance of addictions in your country? Why?

International level

1 Could we talk about the existence of an EU model aligning addiction policies
in Europe?

- If it exists, is it valid to tackle addictions in all EU countries the same way,
or is it necessary to have different models? Why?

2 What are the key elements that can differentiate or unify countries in terms
of drug and addiction policy?

3 What is the main direction of the majority of European countries in drug
policy?

4 Which are the main gaps at international level (UN, EU, WHO, etc.) when
tackling the governance of addictions?

5 What tools do you consider should be enhanced to deal effectively with the
governance of addictions?

Annex 2: Country table template

Country name:

Contextual measures		Country	EU (27)
Total Population[a]	%		
	Total		
Average Age[b]			
GDP per capita[c]	Index EU 100		
	Euros/inhabitant		
Unemployment rate[d]	Total population (%)		
	Under 25 (%)		
Inequality[e]	At-risk poverty rate (2010)[c]		

Framework indicators	Country	EU (27+1)
Esping-Andersen welfare state[f]		
OECD well-being indicators[g]		
Income		
Jobs		
Housing		
Community		
Education		
Environment		
Governance		
Health		
Life satisfaction		
Safety		
Work-life balance		
World Values Survey Index[h]		
TradRat values		
SurvSelf values		
Sustainable Gov. Index[i]		
Status index		
Management index		
Corruption Perception Index[j]		

Annex 2: (continued) Country table template

Consumption measures			
		Country	**EU (27+1)**
Alcohol: Average adult (15+) per capita consumption in litres[k]	Recorded		
	Recorded + unrecorded		
Tobacco[l]	% of smokers		
	Cigarettes per day		
Cannabis annual prevalence[m]	All adults 15–64		
	Young adults 15–34		
	Youth 15–24		
Heroin: prevalence of injecting drug use (overall type of drug use, rate/1000)[n]	Lower		
	Upper		
Primary drug abuse among persons treated[o]	Cannabis		
	Opioids		

Geopolitics of drugs
Position in a drug traffic route (gateway, traffic, transhipment point, final destination)[p]
Major drug traffic[q]

Policy measures[r]		
Previous national strategy (year, main focus)		
Previous national action plan (year, main actors)		
Current national strategy (year, main focus and differences between the last)		
Current national plan (year, main focus and differences between the last)		
Accountability (presence and direction)		
Information availability (presence and language)		
Ministry responsible		
Ministries involved		
Budget specificities (information transparency, clearness and % of government's budget)[j]		
Specific coordination organism		
Definition of addictions		
Specific law and regulation (presence/absence and changes over time, main objective)	Alcohol	
	Tobacco	
	Illicit drugs	

Annex 2: (continued) Country table template

		Country	EU
Public-private collaboration (presence/absence; type [prevention, treatment, etc.]; main actors)	General		
	Alcohol		
	Tobacco		
	Illicit Drugs		
Policy planning (decentralization: y/n)			
Implementation (decentralizations: y/n)			
Classification of drugs	Main laws and lists of substances		
	Classification determines penalty		
	Application of laws		
Illicit consumption of drugs	Legal basis and definition of offence		
	Penalty established		
Illicit possession of drugs	Description		
	Basic possession offences and penalties		
Illicit drug trafficking	Penalties (imprisonment)		
	User-dealers difference		
Best practices[s]			
General (year, drug governance, type)			
Substance specific (year, type: prevention, treatment, etc.)	Alcohol		
	Tobacco		
	Cannabis		
	Heroin		
Media coverage			
Policy timeline			

[a] Source: percentage and total data from Eurostat, *Member countries of the European Union,* 2011, Copyright © European Union, 1995–2013, available from http://europa.eu/about-eu/countries/member-countries/index_en.htm.

[b] Source: data from Eurostat, *Population structure and ageing,* 2012, Copyright © European Union, 1995–2013, available from http://epp.eurostat.ec.europa.eu/statistics_explained/index.php/Population_structure_and_ageing.

Annex 2: (continued) Country table template

c Source: Eurostat, *GDP per capita—annual data,* Copyright © European Union, 1995–2013, available from http://appsso.eurostat.ec.europa.eu/nui/show.do?dataset=nama_aux_gph&lang=en.

d Source: total population data from EUROSTAT, *Unemployment rate by sex and age groups—annual average, %,* Copyright © European Union, 1995–2013, available from http://appsso.eurostat. ec.europa.eu/nui/show.do?dataset=une_rt_a&lang=e; Youth data from EUROSTAT, *Unemployment rate by age group,* Copyright © European Union, 1995–2013, available from http://epp.eurostat. ec.europa.eu/tgm/table.do?tab=table&init=1&plugin=1&language=en&pcode=tsdec460.

e Source: data from Eurostat, *At-risk-of-poverty rate by sex,* Copyright © European Union, 1995–2013, available from http://epp.eurostat.ec.europa.eu/tgm/table.do?tab=table&init=1&plugin=1&language= en&pcode=tessi010.

f Source: data from Esping-Andersen, G., *The three worlds of welfare capitalism,* Polity Press, Oxford, UK, Copyright © 1990.

g Source: data from Organisation for Economic Cooperation and Development (OECD), *OECD Better Life Index,* Copyright OECD, available from http://www.oecdbetterlifeindex.org.

h Source: data from *World Values Survey,* Copyright © 2012 World Values Survey, available from http:// www.worldvaluessurvey.org/index_html.

i Source: Status index data from Sustainable Government Indications 2011 (SGI), *Status Index,* Copyright © Bertelsmann Stiftung 2011, available from http://www.sgi-network.org/index.php?page=index& index=status; Management index data from Sustainable Government Indications 2011 (SGI), *Management Index,* Copyright © Bertelsmann Stiftung 2011, available from http://www.sgi-network. org/index.php?page=index&index=management.

j Source: data from Transparency International, *Corruption Perceptions Index* 2011, Copyright © Transparency International, 2013 http://www.transparency.org/cpi2011/results.

k Source: recorded data from Global Health Observatory Data Repository, *Levels of Consumption: Recorded adult per capita consumption, from 1961, Total by country,* Copyright © World Health Organization (WHO) 2013, available from http://apps.who.int/gho/data/node.main.A1025?lang=en? showonly=GISAH; Recorded and unrecorded data from Global Health Observatory Data Repository, *Levels of Consumption: Unrecorded adult per capita consumption by country,* Copyright © World Health Organization (WHO) 2013, available from http://apps.who.int/gho/data/node.main.A1034? lang=en.

l Source: percentage of smokers' data from Eurostat, *Daily smokers of cigarettes by sex, age and educational attainment level (%),* Copyright © European Union, 1995–2013, available from http://appsso. eurostat.ec.europa.eu/nui/show.do?dataset=hlth_ehis_de3&lang=en; Cigarettes per day data from European Commission, *Eurobarometer 72.3: Tobacco,* Special Eurobarometer 332, Copyright © 2009, available from http://ec.europa.eu/public_opinion/archives/ebs/ebs_332_en.pdf.

m Source: all adults 15–64 data from European Monitoring Centre for Drugs and Drug Addiction (EMCD-DA), Table GPS-2. *Last 12 months prevalence of drug use by age and country, most recent national general population survey available since 2000, Part (i) All adults (aged 15–64),* Copyright © EMCDDA, 1995–2012, available from http://www.emcdda.europa.eu/stats13#display:/stats13/gpstab2a; Young adults 15–34 data from European Monitoring Centre for Drugs and Drug Addiction (EMCDDA), Table GPS-2. *Last 12 months prevalence of drug use by age and country, most recent national general population survey available since 2000, Part (ii) Young adults (15–34),* Copyright © EMCDDA, 1995–2012, available from http://www.emcdda.europa.eu/stats13#display:/stats13/gpstab2b; and Youth 15–24 data from European Monitoring Centre for Drugs and Drug Addiction (EMCDDA), Table GPS-2. *Last 12 months prevalence of drug use by age and country, most recent national general population survey available since 2000, Part (iii) Youth (aged 15–24),* Copyright © EMCDDA, 1995–2012, available from http://www.emcdda.europa.eu/stats13#display:/stats13/gpstab2c.

n Source: data from European Monitoring Centre for Drugs and Drug Addiction (EMCDDA), Table PDU-1. *Estimates of prevalence of problem drug use at national level: summary table, 2006–11, rate per 1 000 aged 15–64, Part (iii) Problem opioid use,* Copyright © EMCDDA, 1995–2012, available from http://www.emcdda.europa.eu/stats13#display:/stats13/pdutab1c.

Annex 2: (continued) Country table template

[o] Source: National Reports. These include national strategies, national action plans, laws, regulations and EMCDDA national reports.

[p] Source: data from Central Intelligence Agency (CIA), *The World Factbook 2013–14, CIA,* Washington, DC, USA, available from https://www.cia.gov/library/publications/the-world-factbook/index.html.

[q] Source: data from Central Intelligence Agency (CIA), *The World Factbook 2013–14, CIA,* Washington, DC, USA, available from https://www.cia.gov/library/publications/the-world-factbook/index.html.

[r] Source: National Reports. These include national strategies, national action plans, laws, regulations and EMCDDA national reports.

[s] Source: data from European Monitoring Centre for Drugs and Drug Addiction (EMCDDA), *Best Practice Portal,* Copyright © EMCDDA, 1995–2012, available from http://www.emcdda.europa.eu/best-practice.

Annex 3: Operationalization of variables for the cluster analysis

Here we present the ten variables used to capture whether a country has a well-being and relational management approach or a safety and disease approach:

◆ Ministry of Health: Is the Ministry of Health responsible for drug and addiction policies? ($Y = 1 \mid N = 0$).

  • If the Ministry of Health is the institution responsible for tackling drug and addiction issues, this represents a public-health approach. This contrasts with those countries that give this responsibility to other ministries, such as the Ministry of the Interior, which would represent having a safety and disease rather than a public-health approach.

◆ Classification determines penalties: Does drug classification determine penalties? ($Y = 1 \mid N = 0$).

  • When the legislation of a country takes into account the different levels of risk associated with addictive substances and establishes its penalties according to the level of hazard, it takes into account the multiple facets of this phenomenon and the fact that it cannot be tackled from a single angle. On the other hand, by having the same penalties for all substances, countries are not taking into account recognized practices promoted by international institutions, such as the EU, and address the complexity of legislating addictions and drugs from a single perspective.

◆ Decriminalize possession: Does the country embrace decriminalization policies? ($Y = 1 \mid N = 0$).

  • Decriminalization of possession implies imposing civil penalties, instead of criminal ones, to those possessing illicit substances. Those countries that criminalize drug possession are normally less tolerant and more focused on demand reduction than harm reduction.

◆ Injection rooms (proxy for harm-reduction policies): Does the country have injection rooms? ($Y = 1 \mid N = 0$)

  • Having injection rooms is recognized by experts as an innovative harm-reduction policy. It tries to reduce the social harm that the addicts can cause to society. In this sense, this characteristic also reflects a societal approach that tries to reintegrate addicts into society. Because this measure is adopted by very few countries, it represents the leading countries in the harm-reduction policy domain.

◆ Alcohol policy scales (Karlsson et al. 2012): Does the country rank above the mean for the twenty-eight on the alcohol policy scale? ($Y = 1 \mid N = 0$).

- Tobacco-control scale (Joossens and Raw 2010): Does the country rank above 50 points on a 100-point scale? (Y = 1 | N = 0).
  - Ranking high on the alcohol and tobacco scales means that a country is implementing evidence and research-based regulations, oriented towards reducing the social harm produced by these substances and improving the overall well-being of consumers, addicts, and the population in general. Hence, these countries not only aim to reduce consumption by making it more difficult to buy alcohol and tobacco, but they also pursue improvement of the quality of life. Both scales for legal substances are associated with the protection of the public and society in general.
- Supply reduction in national strategy: Supply reduction is not one of the priorities in the national strategy of the country. (Y = 1 | N = 0).
  - If a country has supply reduction as the first or second priority in its national strategy, it is not prioritizing other demand- and harm-reduction policies more aligned with the public-health approach.
- Public health in national strategy: Does the national strategy have a public-health perspective on its aims? (Y = 1 | N = 0).
- Well-being in national strategy: Does the national strategy have a well-being perspective on its aims? (Y = 1 | N = 0).
  - Placing public health and well-being in the national strategy is a desideratum of the countries wishing to be more aligned with a well-being and relational management approach. However, not all the countries translate this statement of intention into real policies.
- Best practices: Has the country been recognized for having EMCDDA top-ranked best practices? (Y = 1 | N = 0).
  - A country that has best practices with the top rate of the EMCDDA will have a proactive approach to dealing with drugs. Hence, it does not wait until the problem appears but develops the policy proactively. Furthermore, such countries can also be characterized by leading the way in the field of addictions.

The variables presented below have been used to operationalize the structure domain.

- Tackles legal and illicit substances together: Does the country tackle licit and illicit substances together? (Y = 1 | N = 0).
  - By tackling legal and illicit substances together, a government's approach is not focused on dealing with concrete substances but on comprehensively responding to an issue that, although it has many particularities, has a single consequence: addiction.

- Transversality: Ratio of ministries involved in the governance of drugs and addictions (>50% = 1 | <50% = 0).
  - With this indicator we measure the percentage of ministries involved in the design and implementation of addiction policies. When governments involve more than 50 per cent of their ministries in tackling drug and addiction issues, they show a cross-cutting approach that cannot be properly tackled from one single dimension and that requires trans-disciplinarity and collaboration from different policy domains.

- Addiction on objectives: Is the concept of addiction featured in the objectives of the national strategy? (Y = 1 | N = 0).
  - With this variable we measure whether the term 'addiction' appears in the national strategy, meaning the country has a comprehensive view that goes beyond each substance and tries to respond to the overall problem.

- Ad hoc coordinator body: has the country a coordinator or an ad hoc body? (Y = 1 | N = 0).
  - A coordinator ad hoc body is linked to having a comprehensive policy because this body has to coordinate trans-ministerial collaboration and even the participation of non-profit and private stakeholders. This body also has the pivotal function of integrating the visions and efforts of every participant in the policy-making, implementation, and accountability process.

- Non profit organizations in decision-making: Are non-profit organizations involved in the decision-making process? (Y = 1 | N = 0).
  - Including non-profit organizations in the decision-making process means that the government accepts that addiction is an issue that cannot be properly solved without the involvement of third-sector organizations. In many cases, non-profit organizations are implementing drug-related public policies; thus, they are some of the most active actors in the field, with valuable knowledge that could be useful in the decision-making process.

- Businesses in decision-making: Are private organizations involved in the decision-making process? (Y = 1 | N = 0).
  - Similarly, the involvement of businesses in the decision-making process also implies that the executive power acknowledges that the issue will not be solved unless private organizations (including the relevant industry) are involved as a part of the solution. In contrast to non-profit organizations, private institutions are not as involved in the implementation process, but they do have powerful capabilities that can affect the evolution of public policies.

- ◆ Policy-making decentralization: Does this country decentralize policy-making to multi-level governance structures? (Y = 1 | N = 0).

  - By decentralizing policy-making, governments understand that proximity can be a plus to solving drug-related problems. National governments consider that local public institutions play an important role in adjusting the policy to local particularities and needs. Due to their closeness, local public institutions normally have a better knowledge of the problem and can provide a better and more efficient response.

- ◆ Implementation decentralization: Does this country decentralize implementation to multi-level governance structures? (Y = 1 | N = 0)

  - Involving decentralized structures in the implementation process also represents a step towards a comprehensive approach since these decentralized institutions should know the state of the art better and how to deal with the issue. It is worth mentioning that, since most of the countries implement at least one of the policies taken into account, the countries that rate 1 should decentralize implementation for at least two policies (e.g. prevention and harm reduction).

- ◆ Trajectory: How long is the country's experience in the regulation of drugs? (Before the first EU report in 1982 = 1 | After the first EU report = 0).

  - Having a long trajectory in the field of addictions is normally linked to sound policies and continuity. Those countries with longer experience also have more complex structures to face addictions and have learnt many lessons about how to deal with drug-related problems.

Annex 4: Variables codified

Sample table
State factors
Year of entry into the EU
OECD Better Life Initiative
OECD material living conditions
OECD quality of life
Status Index
Management Index
Religion
Traditional vs rational values [−2 to 2]
Survival vs self-expression values [−2 to 2]
Political structure
Corruption Perception Index
Population
GDP per capita
Income level
Unemployment rate
Unemployment rate (youth)
At-risk poverty rate after social transfers
GINI Index
Human Development Index
Policy factors
Location regarding trafficking
Main drug trafficked
Alcohol consumption—recorded
Alcohol consumption—unrecorded
Tobacco consumption—% of smokers
Tobacco consumption—cigarettes per day
Cannabis prevalence all adults 15–64
Cannabis prevalence young adults 15–34
Cannabis prevalence youth 15–24
Heroin prevalence [lower/higher]
FCTC ratification year
Party to the 1961 Single Convention

Annex 4: (continued) Variables codified

Party to the 1961 Single Convention as amended in 1972	
Ratification of 1971 Convention on Psychotropic Substances	
Party to the 1988 Convention	

Strategy

Responsible ministry for drug and addictions policies	Article II.
The drug classification of the country determines the final penalties	
Penalties for possessing drugs are higher than the EU recommendations	
Penalties for trafficking drugs are higher than the EU recommendations	
This country decriminalizes drug possession	
Injection rooms—proxy for harm reduction	
Alcohol policy scale	
Alcohol price	
Adopted written national policy on alcohol	
Tobacco control scale	
Specific national government objectives in tobacco control	
Public health is included in the national strategy	
Well-being is included in the national strategy	
The country has EMCDDA best practices	
Priority in the national strategy	

Structure

Ad hoc organization
Tackles legal and illicit substances together
Number of ministries involved
The country devolves policy-making to decentralized structures
The country devolves implementation to decentralized structures
Non-profit organization in the decision-making
Private organization in the implementation
Addiction is a priority in the national strategy
Year of the first law on illicit substances

Annex 5: Variables for factors construct and their definitions

Variables for state factors construct and their definitions	Source	Year of data collection	Measure
Year of entry into the EU In which of the different years the countries analysed gained the European Union membership	EUROSTAT, *Member countries of the European Union*, 2011, Copyright © European Union, 1995–2013, available from http://europa.eu/about-eu/countries/member-countries/index_en.htm	2012	Year
OECD Better Life Initiative— the OECD Better Life Initiative measures the well-being of people and nations. The OECD has identified 11 dimensions as being essential to well-being, from health and education to local environment, personal security and overall satisfaction with life, as well as more traditional measures such as income, divided in two sub-dimensions: 'material living conditions' and 'quality of life'.	Organisation for Economic Cooperation and Development (OECD), *OECD Better Life Index*, Copyright OECD, available from http://www.oecdbetterlifeindex.org	2011/2012	Scale: from 0 being total absence of well-being to 10 maximum well-being
OECD material living conditions Within this set of indicators allocated in the Better Life Initiative index one can find: Housing, Income, Jobs, Environment and Safety	Organisation for Economic Cooperation and Development (OECD), *OECD Better Life Index*, Copyright OECD, available from http://www.oecdbetterlifeindex.org	2011/2012	Scale: from 0 being total absence of material living conditions to 10 maximum comfort in material living conditions.
OECD quality of life Within this set of indicators allocated in the Better Life Initiative Index one can find: Community, Education, Civic engagement, health, Life satisfaction, work-life balance.	Organisation for Economic Cooperation and Development (OECD), *OECD Better Life Index*, Copyright OECD, available from http://www.oecdbetterlifeindex.org	2011/2012	Scale: from 0 being total absence of quality of life to 10 maximum perception of quality of life

continued

Annex 5: (continued) Variables for factors construct and their definitions

Variables for state factors construct and their definitions	Source	Year of data collection	Measure
Status Index— the Sustainable Governance Indicators (SGI) project is a cross-national survey of governance in the OECD that identifies reform needs and highlights forward-looking practices. The Status Index examines states' reform needs in terms of the quality of democracy and performance in policy fields in five dimensions: democracy (state of democratic institutions); economy and employment (how economic policies address globalization); social affairs (whether social policies facilitate an equal and fair society); security (to what extent security policies protect citizens); and resources (how policies address issues of sustainability).	Sustainable Government Indications 2011 (SGI), *Status Index*, Copyright © Bertelsmann Stiftung 2011, available from http://www.sgi-network.org/index.php?page=index&index=status	2011/2012	Scale: from 0 being no effective policies for citizens needs to 10 maximum effective policies
Management Index— from the SGI. The Management Index focuses on governance capacities in terms of steering capability and accountability in four dimensions: steering capability (whether the government has steering capabilities); policy implementation (whether the government implements policies effectively); institutional learning (whether the government adapts to internal and external developments); and accountability (to what extent non-governmental actors are involved in policy-making).	Sustainable Government Indications 2011 (SGI), *Status Index*, Copyright © Bertelsmann Stiftung 2011, available from http://www.sgi-network.org/index.php?page=index&index=status	2011/2012	Scale: from 0 being no governance capacities to 10 maximum governance capacities

Religion— percentage of major religious belief of the country	CIA, *The world factbook 2013–14*, CIA, Washington, DC, USA, available from <https://www.cia.gov/library/publications/the-world-factbook/index.html>	Differ for each country (latest available)/2012	Scale: no scale, the name of major religion
Traditional vs rational values— a dimension used in the World Values Surveys study designed to provide a comprehensive measurement of all major areas of human concern, from religion to politics to economic and social life. This particular dimension reflects the contrast between societies in which religion is very important and those in which it is not. A wide range of other orientations are closely linked with this dimension. Societies close to the traditional pole emphasize the importance of parent-child ties and deference to authority, along with absolute standards and traditional family values, and reject divorce, abortion, euthanasia, and suicide. These societies have high levels of national pride, and a nationalistic outlook. Societies with secular-rational values have the opposite preferences on all of these topics	World Values Survey, Copyright © 2012 World Values Survey, available from http://www.worldvaluessurvey.crg/index_html	Differ for each country (latest available)/2012	Scale: from −2 being traditional values to +2 being rational values

continued

Annex 5: (continued) Variables for factors construct and their definitions

Variables for state factors construct and their definitions	Source	Year of data collection	Measure
Survival vs self-expression values— a dimension used in the World Values Surveys study designed to provide a comprehensive measurement of all major areas of human concern, from religion to politics to economic and social life. This particular dimension is linked with the transition from industrial society to post-industrial society—which brings a polarization between survival and self-expression values. The unprecedented wealth that has accumulated in advanced societies during the past generation means that an increasing share of the population has grown up taking survival for granted. Thus, priorities have shifted from an overwhelming emphasis on economic and physical security towards an increasing emphasis on subjective well-being, self-expression, and quality of life.	World Values Survey, Copyright © 2012 World Values Survey, available from http://www.worldvaluessurvey.org/index_html	Differ for each country (latest available)/2012	Scale: from −2 being survival values to +2 being self-expression values
Political structure— typology of governmental structure. Refers to institutions or groups and their relation to each other, their patterns of interaction within political systems, and to political regulations, laws and the norms present in political systems in such a way that they constitute the political landscape of the political entity.	Central Intelligence Agency (CIA), *The world factbook 2013–14*, CIA, Washington, DC, USA, available from <https://www.cia.gov/library/publications/the-world-factbook/index.html>	Differ for each country (latest available)/2012	No scale, the name of the type
Corruption Perception Index Scale created by Transparency international—how corrupt the public sectors of the governments are seen to be	Transparency International, *Corruption Perceptions Index 2011*, Copyright © Transparency International, 2013 http://www.transparency.org/cpi2011/results	2011/2012	Scale: from 0 being highly corrupt country to 10 being very clean

Population— percentage of the countries' population within the European Union	Eurostat, *Member countries of the European Union*, 2011, Copyright © European Union, 1995–2013, available from http://europa.eu/about-eu/countries/member-countries/index_en.htm	2011	Percentage
GDP per capita— the volume index of GDP per capita in Purchasing Power Standards (PPS) is expressed in relation to the European Union (EU–27) average set to equal 100. If the index of a country is higher than 100, this country's level of GDP per head is higher than the EU average and vice versa.	Eurostat, *GDP per capita—annual data*, Copyright © European Union, 1995–2013, available from http://appsso.eurostat.ec.europa.eu/nui/show.do?dataset=nama_aux_gph&lang=en	2011	EU 27 is 100
Income level— nominal gross domestic product per capita in euros per inhabitant.	Eurostat, *GDP per capita—annual data*, Copyright © European Union, 1995–2013, available from http://appsso.eurostat.ec.europa.eu/nui/show.do?dataset=nama_aux_gph&lang=en	2011/2011	Euros
Unemployment rate— percentage of unemployed people from the general population	Eurostat, *Unemployment rate by sex and age groups—annual average, %*, Copyright © European Union, 1995–2013, available from http://appsso.eurostat.ec.europa.eu/nui/show.do?dataset=une_rt_a&lang=e	2011	Percentage

continued

Annex 5: (continued) Variables for factors construct and their definitions

Variables for state factors construct and their definitions	Source	Year of data collection	Measure
Unemployment rate (youth)— proportion of unemployed young people from the young population (under 25)	Eurostat, *Unemployment rate by age group*, Copyright © European Union, 1995–2013, available from http://epp.eurostat.ec.europa.eu/tgm/table.do?tab=table&init=1&plugin=1&language=en&pcode=tsdec460	2011	Percentage
At-risk poverty rate after social transfers The share of persons with an equivalized disposable income below the risk-of-poverty threshold, which is set at 60% of the national median equivalized disposable income (after social transfers).	Eurostat, *At-risk-of-poverty rate by sex*, Copyright © European Union, 1995–2013, available from http://epp.eurostat.ec.europa.eu/tgm/table.do?tab=table&init=1&plugin=1&language=en&pcode=tessi010	2011	Percentage
GINI Index— measures the extent to which the distribution of income or consumption expenditure among individuals or households within an economy deviates from a perfectly equal distribution.	The World Bank, *GINI Index*, Copyright © The World Bank Group, available from http://data.worldbank.org/indicator/SI.POV.GINI and Eurostat, *Gini coefficient of equivalized disposable income*, Copyright © European Union, 1995–2013, available from http://appsso.eurostat.ec.europa.eu/nui/show.do?dataset=ilc_di12&lang=en	Differs for each country (latest available)/2011	Scale: 0 represents perfect equality, while an index of 100 implies perfect inequality

Human Development— a composite that combines indicators of life expectancy, educational issues, and income.	United Nations Development Programme, *Country Profiles and International Human Development Indicators*, Copyright © United Nations Development Programme (UNDP), available from http://hdr.undp.org/en/data/profiles/	2011	Measure: composite from 0 to 1. The closer to 1, the higher HDI a country has

Variables for policy factors construct and their definitions

Location regarding trafficking— whether the country is at the beginning, middle, or end of a traffic route, being the entrance, traffic, or final destination of a drug trafficking route.	Central Intelligence Agency (CIA), *The world factbook 2013–14*, CIA, Washington, DC, USA, available from https://www.cia.gov/library/publications/the-world-factbook/index.html	Differ for each country (latest available)/2012	Scale: no scale, which position
Main drug trafficked— which is the most trafficked drug in the country, usually by the number of seizures.	CIA, *The world factbook 2013–14*, CIA, Washington, DC, USA, available from https://www.cia.gov/library/publications/the-world-factbook/index.html	Differ for each country (latest available)/2012	Scale: no scale, name of drug
Alcohol consumption— recorded— recorded adult (15+ years) per capita consumption (in litres of pure alcohol)	Global Health Observatory Data Repository, *Levels of consumption: Recorded adult per capita consumption, from 1961, total by country*, Copyright © World Health Organization (WHO) 2013, available from http://apps.who.int/gho/data/node.main.A1025?lang=en?showonly=GISAH;	2005/2012	Litres

continued

Annex 5: (continued) Variables for factors construct and their definitions

Variables for policy factors construct and their definitions

Alcohol consumption— unrecorded— unrecorded adult (15+ years) per capita consumption (in litres of pure alcohol), estimates	Global Health Observatory Data Repository, *Levels of consumption: Unrecorded adult per capita consumption by country,* Copyright © World Health Organization (WHO) 2013, available from http://apps.who.int/gho/data/node.main.A1034?lang=en	2005/2012	Litres
Tobacco consumption— % of smokers— proportion of smokers from the total population	Percentage of smokers' data from Eurostat, *Daily smokers of cigarettes by sex, age and educational attainment level (%),* Copyright © European Union, 1995–2013, available from http://appsso.eurostat.ec.europa.eu/nui/show.do?dataset=hlth_ehis_de3&lang=en	2011	Percentage
Tobacco consumption— cigarettes per day— number of cigarettes per day smoked	European Commission, *Eurobarometer 72.3: Tobacco, Special Eurobarometer 332,* Copyright © 2009, available from. http://ec.europa.eu/public_opinion/archives/ebs/ebs_332_en.pdf	2011	Total number

| Cannabis annual prevalence all adults 15–64—

proportion of the population between 15 and 64 years found to consume cannabis during the year 2011 | European Monitoring Centre for Drugs and Drug Addiction (EMCDDA), *Table GPS–2. Last 12 months prevalence of drug use by age and country, most recent national general population survey available since 2000, Part (i) All adults (aged 15–64),* Copyright © EMCDDA, 1995–2012, available from http://www.emcdda. europa.eu/stats13#display:/stats13/ gpstab2a | 2011 | Percentage |
| Cannabis prevalence young adults 15–34—

the proportion of the population between 15 and 34 years found to consume cannabis during the year 2011 | European Monitoring Centre for Drugs and Drug Addiction (EMCDDA), *Table GPS–2. Last 12 months prevalence of drug use by age and country, most recent national general population survey available since 2000, Part (ii) Young adults (15–34),* Copyright © EMCDDA, 1995–2012, available from http://www.emcdda. europa.eu/stats13#display:/stats13/ gpstab2b | 2011 | Percentage |

continued

Annex 5: (continued) Variables for factors construct and their definitions

Variables for policy factors construct and their definitions

Cannabis prevalence youth 15–24— the proportion of the population between 15 and 24 years found to consume cannabis during the year 2011	European Monitoring Centre for Drugs and Drug Addiction (EMCDDA), Table GPS–2. *Last 12 months prevalence of drug use by age and country, most recent national general population survey available since 2000, Part (iii) Youth (aged 15–24),* Copyright © EMCDDA, 1995–2012, available from http://www.emcdda. europa.eu/stats13#display:/stats13/gpstab2c	2011	Percentage
Heroin prevalence [lower/higher]—estimates about the proportion of the population between 15 and 64 years old for last year use of heroin per 1000 inhabitants. Due to different methods of data collection it has a range between two points: the lowest point and the highest point	European Monitoring Centre for Drugs and Drug Addiction (EMCDDA),Table PDU-1. *Estimates of prevalence of problem drug use at national level: summary table, 2006–11, rate per 1 000 aged 15–64, Part (iii) Problem opioid use,* Copyright © EMCDDA, 1995–2012, available from http://www.emcdda.europa.eu/stats13#display:/stats13/pdutab1c	2011	A number per 1000 inhabitants

continued

	Year of ratification		

FCTC (Framework Convention for Tobacco Control) ratification year—the WHO FCTC treaty was adopted in 2003. Its main objective is 'to protect present and future generations from the devastating health, social, environmental and economic consequences of tobacco consumption and exposure to tobacco smoke by providing a framework for tobacco control measures to be implemented by the Parties at the national, regional and international levels in order to reduce continually and substantially the prevalence of tobacco use and exposure to tobacco smoke' (WHO FCTC, WHO Framework Convention On Tobacco Control, Article 3, p. 5, Copyright © World Health Organization 2003)

WHO Framework Convention on Tobacco Control (WHO FCTC), Copyright © World Health Organization 2013, available from http://www.who.int/fctc/en — 2011

Party to the 1961 Single Convention on Narcotic Drugs UN Convention adopted in 1961. The Convention aims 'to combat drug abuse by coordinated international action. There are two forms of intervention and control that work together. First, it seeks to limit the possession, use, trade in, distribution, import, export, manufacture and production of drugs exclusively to medical and scientific purposes. Second, it combats drug trafficking through international cooperation to deter and discourage drug traffickers' (UN, Single Convention on Narcotic Drugs, 1961, as amended by the 1972 Protocol Amending the Single Convention on Narcotic Drugs, 1961, Copyright © 1961 and 1972, available at https://www.unodc.org/pdf/convention_1961_en.pdf)

United Nations Drug Control Programme and the Centre for International Crime Prevention (UNODC), *Treaties*, Copyright © 2013 UNODC, available from http://treaties.un.org/Pages/ViewDetails.aspx?src=TREATY&mtdsg_no=VI-18&chapter=6&lang=en — 2011

Annex 5: (continued) Variables for factors construct and their definitions

Variables for policy factors construct and their definitions		
Party to the 1961 Single Convention as amended in 1972—	United Nations Drug Control Programme and the Centre for International Crime Prevention (UNODC), *Treaties*, Copyright © 2013 UNODC, available from http://www.unodc.org/unod/en/treaties/index.html?ref=menuside	2011 Year
the 1972 Protocol Amending the Single Convention on Narcotic Drugs made several changes. It highlighted the need for treatment and rehabilitation of drug addicts, instructing parties to take 'all practicable measures for the prevention of abuse of psychotropic substances and for the early identification, treatment, education, after-care, rehabilitation, and social reintegration of the persons involved'. It also expanded the International Narcotics Control Board from 11 members to 13 members (United Nations, Single Convention on Narcotic Drugs, 1961, as amended by the 1972 Protocol Amending the Single Convention on Narcotic Drugs, 1961, Article 35, p. 19, Copyright © United nations 1972)		
Ratification of 1971 Convention on Psychotropic Substances—	United Nations Drug Control Programme and the Centre for International Crime Prevention (UNODC), *Treaties*, Copyright © 2013 UNODC, available from http://www.unodc.org/unod/en/treaties/index.html?ref=menuside>	2011 Year
the Convention on Psychotropic Substances of 1971 is a UN treaty designed to control psychoactive drugs such as amphetamines, barbiturates, benzodiazepines, and psychedelics; it was signed in Vienna, Austria on 21 February 1971		
Party to the 1988 Convention—	United Nations Drug Control Programme and the Centre for International Crime Prevention (UNODC), *Treaties*, Copyright © 2013 UNODC, available from http://www.unodc.org/unod/en/treaties/index.html?ref=menuside	2011 Year
the UN Convention Against Illicit Traffic in Narcotic Drugs and Psychotropic Substances of 1988 is one of three major drug control treaties currently in force. It provides additional legal mechanisms for enforcing the 1961 Single Convention on Narcotic Drugs and the 1971 Convention on Psychotropic Substances. The Convention entered into force on 11 November 1990. As of 1 February 2013, there were 188 Parties to the Convention		

Public spending on drug-related activities as a percentage of GDP— estimate of national public spending on illicit drug-related activities as a percentage of GDP	European Monitoring Centre for Drugs and Drug Addiction (EMCDDA), *Countries: national drug-related information and data*, Copyright © EMCDDA, 1995–2012, available from http://www.emcdda.europa.eu/countries/public-expenditure	From 2006 to 2011 (depending on the case)	Percentage

Variables for the strategy construct and their definitions

Responsible ministry for drug and addictions policies— main national institution responsible for governing drugs and addictions	National reports	2011	Qualitative data
The drug classification of the country determines the final penalties— the indicator determines whether a country's legislation takes into account the risk that different substances pose to individuals and society	National reports	2011	Yes/No
Penalties for possessing drugs are higher than the EU recommendations— whether a country has stricter penalties for possession than the ones provided by the Council of the EU	*Council of the EU Framework Decision 2004/757/JHA of 25 October 2004 laying down minimum provisions on the constituent elements of criminal acts and penalties in the field of illicit drug trafficking*, available from http://db.eurocrim.org/db/en/doc/247.pdf	2011	Yes/No

continued

Annex 5: (continued) Variables for factors construct and their definitions

Variables for the strategy construct and their definitions

Penalties for trafficking drugs are higher than the EU recommendations— whether a country has stricter penalties for trafficking than the ones provided by the Council of the EU	*Council of the EU Framework Decision 2004/757/JHA of 25 October 2004 laying down minimum provisions on the constituent elements of criminal acts and penalties in the field of illicit drug trafficking*, available from http://db.eurocrim.org/db/en/doc/247.pdf	2011	Yes/No
This country decriminalizes drug possession— whether the country has decriminalized the possession of illicit substances, either cannabis or heroin or both	National reports	2011	Yes/No
Injection rooms—proxy for harm reduction— whether a country has or does not have injection rooms as an innovative harm-reduction policy.	National reports	2011	Yes/No
Alcohol policy scale— scale measuring the strictness and comprehensiveness of formal alcohol policies	Karlsson, T. et al., Does alcohol policy make any difference? Scales and consumption, in P. Anderson et al. (eds), *Alcohol policy in Europe: Evidence from AMPHORA*, The AMPHORA project, Copyright © 2012, available from www.amphoraproject.net/view.php?id_cont=45	2012	38.5–133

Alcohol price— price level indices for alcoholic beverages being EU27 = 100	EUROSTAT. *Purchasing power parties (PPPs), price level indices and real expenditures for ESA95 aggregates*, Copyright © European Union, 1995–2013, available from http://appsso.eurostat.ec.europa.eu/nui/show.do?dataset=prc_ppp_ind&lang=en	2009/2011	0–234
Adopted written national policy on alcohol— whether or not a country has specific national strategies to deal with alcohol and its consequences	National reports	2011	Yes/No
Tobacco Control Scale— quantifies the implementation of tobacco control policies at country level, and is based on policies which prioritize a comprehensive tobacco control programme. These are: price, bans/restrictions, information, advertising, warning labels, and treatment	Joossens, L. and Raw, M., *The Tobacco Control Scale 2010 in Europe*, Association of the European Cancer Leagues, Belgium, Copyright © 2010	2010	0–100
Specific national government objectives in tobacco control— whether a country has specific national strategies to deal with tobacco and its consequences or not	National reports	2011	Yes/No
Public health is included in the national strategy— whether the national strategy includes public health as one of its top priorities	National strategies	2011	Yes/No
Well-being is included in the national strategy— whether the national strategy includes well-being as one of its top priorities	National strategies.	2011	Yes/No

continued

Annex 5: (continued) Variables for factors construct and their definitions

Variables for the strategy construct and their definitions

Variable	Source	Year	Measurement
The country has EMCDDA best practices— presents if a country has best practices as reported by the EMCDDA or not. 0 means that the country does not have EMCDDA best practices. From 1 to 3 the country has best practices, 3 being the maximum score possible. The policies taken into account are: harm reduction, prevention, treatment, social reintegration, and interventions in the criminal justice systems	European Monitoring Centre for Drugs and Drug Addiction (EMCDDA), *Best practice portal*, Copyright © EMCDDA, 1995–2012, available from http://www.emcdda.europa.eu/best-practice	2011	0–3
Priority in the national strategy— indicates, according to each national strategy, which is the top policy priority	National strategies	2011	Qualitative

Variables for the structure construct and their definitions

Variable	Source	Year	Measurement
Ad hoc organization— whether a country has a special body in charge of the coordination of the governance of drugs and addictions	National reports	2011	Yes/No
Tackles legal and illicit substances together— the indicators present if a country tackles legal (i.e. alcohol or tobacco) and illicit substances with a single national approach	National strategies	2011	Yes/No
Number of ministries involved— indicates the number of ministries involved in the governance of addictions, over the total ministries of the country.	National reports	2011	Percentage

continued

The country decentralizes policy-making— whether a country devolves the policy-making of at least more than one of its drug-related policy measures to decentralized structures (i.e. regions, federal states, municipalities, etc.)	National reports	2011	Yes/No
The country decentralizes implementation to decentralized structures— whether a country devolves the implementation of at least more than one of its drug-related policy measures to decentralized structures (i.e. regions, federal states, municipalities, etc.)	National reports	2011	Yes/No
Non-profit organization in the decision-making— whether a country involves non-profit organizations in the decision-making process	National reports	2011	Yes/No
Private organization in the implementation— whether a country involves non-profit organizations in the implementation process	National reports	2011	Yes/No
Addiction is a priority in the national strategy— the indicator takes into account whether the national strategy includes well-being as one of its top priorities	National strategies	2011	Yes/No
Year of the first law on illicit substances— year in which the first law aimed at tackling illicit substances was passed	European Monitoring Centre for Drugs and Drug Addiction (EMCDDA), Country legal profiles, Copyright © EMCDDA, 1995–2012, available from http://www.emcdda.europa.eu/html.cfm/index5174EN.html?pluginMethod=eldd.countryprofiles&country	2011	Year

Annex 6: Austria—model 3

State factors

Year of entry into the EU	1995
OECD Better Life Initiative	7/10
OECD material living conditions	6.45/10
OECD quality of life	7.53/10
Status Index	6.86/10
Management Index	6.39/10
Majority religion	Catholicism
Traditional vs rational values [–2 to 2]	0.25
Survival vs self-expression values [–2 to 2]	1.43
Political structure	Federal
Corruption Perception Index	8
Population	1.65
GDP per capita	129
Income level	35,700
Unemployment rate	4.2
Unemployment rate (youth)	8.3
At risk poverty rate after social transfers	12.1
GINI Index	26.3
Human Development Index	0.9

Policy factors

Location regarding trafficking	Transhipment point for heroin and cocaine
Main drug trafficked	Cannabis
Alcohol consumption—recorded	12.6
Alcohol consumption—unrecorded	13.24
Tobacco consumption—% of smokers	34
Tobacco consumption—cigarettes per day	17.7
Cannabis prevalence all adults 15–64	3.5
Cannabis prevalence young adults 15–34	6.6
Cannabis prevalence youth 15–24	10.6
Heroin prevalence [lower/higher]	2.19/4.19
FCTC ratification year	2005
Party to the 1961 Single Convention	1961

Annex 6: (continued) Austria—model 3

Party to the 1961 Single Convention as amended in 1972	1978
Ratification of 1971 Convention on Psychotropic Substances	1997
Party to the 1988 Convention	1989
National public spending on drug-related activities—% of GDP	n.a.

Strategy

Responsible ministry for drug and addictions policies	Ministry of Health
The drug classification of the country determines the final penalties	No
Penalties for possessing drugs are higher than the EU recommendations	No
Penalties for trafficking drugs are higher than the EU recommendations	Yes
This country decriminalizes drug possession	No
Injection rooms—proxy for harm reduction	No
Alcohol policy scale	40
Alcohol price	95
Adopted written national policy on alcohol	Yes
Tobacco control scale	32
Specific national government objectives in tobacco control	No
Public health is included in the national strategy	No
Well-being is included in the national strategy	No
The country has EMCDDA best practices	1 & 2
Priority in the national strategy	Prevention

Structure

Ad hoc organization	No
Tackles legal and illicit substances together	No
Number of ministries involved	12/12
The country devolves policy-making to decentralized structures	Yes
The country devolves implementation to decentralized structures	Yes
Non-profit organization in the decision-making	No
Private organization in the implementation	No
Addiction is a priority in the national strategy	Yes
Year of the first law on illicit substances	1951

Data source: see Annex 5: Variables for factors construct and their definitions.

Annex 7: Belgium—model 1

State factors

Year of entry into the EU	1952
OECD Better Life Initiative	7.19/10
OECD material living conditions	6.86/10
OECD quality of life	7.53/10
Status Index	7.17/10
Management Index	6/10
Majority religion	Catholicism
Traditional vs rational values [–2 to 2]	0.5
Survival vs self-expression values [–2 to 2]	1.13
Political structure	Federal
Corruption Perception Index	7.1/10
Population	2.15%
GDP per capita	129
Income level	35,700
Unemployment rate	7.2
Unemployment rate (youth)	18.7
At risk poverty rate after social transfers	14.6
GINI Index	26.3
Human Development Index	0.9

Policy factors

Location regarding trafficking	Transhipment point. Producer of synthetic drugs
Main drug trafficked	Cannabis
Alcohol consumption—recorded	9.8
Alcohol consumption—unrecorded	10.77
Tobacco consumption—% of smokers	30%
Tobacco consumption—cigarettes per day	15.7
Cannabis prevalence all adults 15–64	5.1
Cannabis prevalence young adults 15–34	11.2
Cannabis prevalence youth 15–24	11.9
Heroin prevalence [lower/higher]	3.46/4.19
FCTC ratification year	2005
Party to the 1961 Single Convention	1961

Annex 7: (continued) Belgium—model 1

Party to the 1961 Single Convention as amended in 1972	1984
Ratification of 1971 Convention on Psychotropic Substances	1995
Party to the 1988 Convention	1989
National public spending on drug-related activities—% of GDP	0.11%

Strategy

Responsible ministry for drug and addictions policies	Ministry of Health
The drug classification of the country determines the final penalties	Yes
Penalties for possessing drugs are higher than the EU recommendations	No
Penalties for trafficking drugs are higher than the EU recommendations	Yes
This country decriminalizes drug possession	Yes
Injection rooms—proxy for harm reduction	No
Alcohol policy scale	53/133
Alcohol price	101/234
Adopted written national policy on alcohol	No
Tobacco control scale	50/100
Specific national government objectives in tobacco control	Yes
Public health is included in the national strategy	No
Well-being is included in the national strategy	Yes
The country has EMCDDA best practices	1, 2 & 3
Priority in the national strategy	Prevention

Structure

Ad hoc organization	Yes
Tackles legal and illicit substances together	Yes
Number of ministries involved	12/12
The country devolves policy-making to decentralized structures	Yes
The country devolves implementation to decentralized structures	Yes
Non-profit organization in the decision-making	No
Private organization in the implementation	No
Addiction is a priority in the national strategy	No
Year of the first law on illicit substances	1921

Data source: see Annex 5: Variables for factors construct and their definitions.

Annex 8: Bulgaria—model 3

State factors	
Year of entry into the EU	2007
OECD Better Life Initiative	–
OECD material living conditions	–
OECD quality of life	–
Status Index	–
Management Index	–
Majority religion	Orthodoxy
Traditional vs rational values [–2 to 2]	1.13
Survival vs self-expression values [–2 to 2]	–1.01
Political structure	Unitary
Corruption Perception Index	3.6/10
Population	1.48%
GDP per capita	45
Income level	4,800
Unemployment rate	11.2%
Unemployment rate (youth)	26.6%
At risk poverty rate after social transfers	20.7%
GINI Index	33.2
Human Development Index	0.8
Policy factors	
Location regarding trafficking	European gateway for Balkan route
Main drug trafficked	Heroin
Alcohol consumption—recorded	11.2
Alcohol consumption—unrecorded	12.44
Tobacco consumption—% of smokers	30%
Tobacco consumption—cigarettes per day	15.8
Cannabis prevalence all adults 15–64	2.7
Cannabis prevalence young adults 15–34	6
Cannabis prevalence youth 15–24	8.7
Heroin prevalence [lower/higher]	–
FCTC ratification year	2005
Party to the 1961 Single Convention	1996

Annex 8: (continued) Bulgaria—model 3

Party to the 1961 Single Convention as amended in 1972	1996
Ratification of 1971 Convention on Psychotropic Substances	1972
Party to the 1988 Convention	1992
National public spending on drug-related activities—% of GDP	n.a.

Strategy

Responsible ministry for drug and addictions policies	Ministry of Health
The drug classification of the country determines the final penalties	No
Penalties for possessing drugs are higher than the EU recommendations	Yes
Penalties for trafficking drugs are higher than the EU recommendations	Yes
This country decriminalizes drug possession	No
Injection rooms—proxy for harm reduction	No
Alcohol policy scale	52/133
Alcohol price	77/234
Adopted written national policy on alcohol	No
Tobacco control scale	40/100
Specific national government objectives in tobacco control	Yes
Public health is included in the national strategy	No
Well-being is included in the national strategy	Yes
The country has EMCDDA best practices	No
Priority in the national strategy	Demand reduction

Structure

Ad hoc organization	Yes
Tackles legal and illicit substances together	Yes
Number of ministries involved	11/15
The country devolves policy-making to decentralized structures	No
The country devolves implementation to decentralized structures	Yes
Non-profit organization in the decision-making	No
Private organization in the implementation	No
Addiction is a priority in the national strategy	No
Year of the first law on illicit substances	1990

Data source: See Annex 5: Variables for factors construct and their definitions.

Annex 9: Cyprus—model 3

State factors	
Year of entry into the EU	2004
OECD Better Life Initiative	–
OECD material living conditions	–
OECD quality of life	–
Status Index	–
Management Index	–
Majority religion	Catholicism
Traditional vs rational values [–2 to 2]	–0.56
Survival vs self-expression values [–2 to 2]	0.013
Political structure	Unitary
Corruption Perception Index	6.3/10
Population	0.16%
GDP per capita	92
Income level	21,100
Unemployment rate	7.8%
Unemployment rate (youth)	22.4%
At risk poverty rate after social transfers	15.8%
GINI Index	29.1
Human Development Index	0.8
Policy factors	
Location regarding trafficking	Transit and final destination
Main drug trafficked	Cannabis and heroin
Alcohol consumption—recorded	8.3
Alcohol consumption—unrecorded	9.3
Tobacco consumption—% of smokers	23.9%
Tobacco consumption—cigarettes per day	21.7
Cannabis prevalence all adults 15–64	4.4
Cannabis prevalence young adults 15–34	7.9
Cannabis prevalence youth 15–24	7.5
Heroin prevalence [lower/higher]	3/-
FCTC ratification year	2005
Party to the 1961 Single Convention	–
Party to the 1961 Single Convention as amended in 1972	–

Annex 9: (continued) Cyprus—model 3

Ratification of 1971 Convention on Psychotropic Substances	–
Party to the 1988 Convention	–
National public spending on drug-related activities—% of GDP	0.04%

Strategy

Responsible ministry for drug and addictions policies	Ministry of Health
The drug classification of the country determines the final penalties	Yes
Penalties for possessing drugs are higher than the EU recommendations	Yes
Penalties for trafficking drugs are higher than the EU recommendations	Yes
This country decriminalizes drug possession	No
Injection rooms—proxy for harm reduction	No
Alcohol policy scale	70/133
Alcohol price	119/234
Adopted written national policy on alcohol	Yes
Tobacco control scale	40/100
Specific national government objectives in tobacco control	No
Public health is included in the national strategy	No
Well-being is included in the national strategy	No
The country has EMCDDA best practices	1 & 2
Priority in the national strategy	Prevention

Structure

Ad hoc organization	Yes
Tackles legal and illicit substances together	No
Number of ministries involved	6/12
The country devolves policy-making to decentralized structures	No
The country devolves implementation to decentralized structures	No
Non-profit organization in the decision-making	No
Private organization in the implementation	No
Addiction is a priority in the national strategy	No
Year of the first law on illicit substances	1977

Data source: see Annex 5: Variables for factors construct and their definitions.

Annex 10: Czech Republic—model 1

State factors

Year of entry into the EU	2004
OECD Better Life Initiative	5.47/10
OECD material living conditions	4.23/10
OECD quality of life	6.71/10
Status Index	6.78/10
Management Index	5.88/10
Majority religion	Catholicism
Traditional vs rational values [−2 to 2]	1.23
Survival vs self-expression values [−2 to 2]	0.38
Political structure	Regionalized
Corruption Perception Index	4.6/10
Population	2.07%
GDP per capita	80
Income level	14,900
Unemployment rate	6.7%
Unemployment rate (youth)	18%
At risk poverty rate after social transfers	9%
GINI Index	25.2
Human Development Index	0.9

Policy factors

Location regarding trafficking	Transhipment point and synthetic drugs producer
Main drug trafficked	Cannabis
Alcohol consumption—recorded	15
Alcohol consumption—unrecorded	16.45
Tobacco consumption—% of smokers	24.9%
Tobacco consumption—cigarettes per day	13.9
Cannabis prevalence all adults 15–64	11.1
Cannabis prevalence young adults 15–34	21.6
Cannabis prevalence youth 15–24	29.5
Heroin prevalence [lower/higher]	3.68/4.6
FCTC ratification year	Not ratified
Party to the 1961 Single Convention	1993

Annex 10: (continued) Czech Republic—model 1

Party to the 1961 Single Convention as amended in 1972	1993
Ratification of 1971 Convention on Psychotropic Substances	1993
Party to the 1988 Convention	1993
National public spending on drug-related activities—% of GDP	0.17%

Strategy

Responsible ministry for drug and addictions policies	Prime minister
The drug classification of the country determines the final penalties	Yes
Penalties for possessing drugs are higher than the EU recommendations	No
Penalties for trafficking drugs are higher than the EU recommendations	Yes
This country decriminalizes drug possession	Yes
Injection rooms—proxy for harm reduction	No
Alcohol policy scale	64/133
Alcohol price	89/234
Adopted written national policy on alcohol	Yes
Tobacco control scale	34/100
Specific national government objectives in tobacco control	Yes
Public health is included in the national strategy	No
Well-being is included in the national strategy	No
The country has EMCDDA best practices	1
Priority in the national strategy	Prevention

Structure

Ad hoc organization	Yes
Tackles legal and illicit substances together	Yes
Number of ministries involved	13/13
The country devolves policy-making to decentralized structures	Yes
The country devolves implementation to decentralized structures	Yes
Non-profit organization in the decision-making	Yes
Private organization in the implementation	Yes
Addiction is a priority in the national strategy	Yes
Year of the first law on illicit substances	1962

Data source: see Annex 5: Variables for factors construct and their definitions.

Annex 11: Denmark—model 3

State factors

Year of entry into the EU	1973
OECD Better Life Initiative	7.2/10
OECD material living conditions	5.9/10
OECD quality of life	8.5/10
Status Index	8.34/10
Management Index	7.9/10
Majority religion	Protestantism
Traditional vs rational values [–2 to 2]	1.16
Survival vs self-expression values [–2 to 2]	1.87
Political structure	Unitary
Corruption Perception Index	9.4/10
Population	1.09%
GDP per capita	125
Income level	43,200
Unemployment rate	7.6%
Unemployment rate (youth)	14.2%
At risk poverty rate after social transfers	13.3%
GINI Index	27.8
Human Development Index	0.9

Policy factors

Location regarding trafficking	Transit and final destination
Main drug trafficked	Cannabis
Alcohol consumption—recorded	11.4
Alcohol consumption—unrecorded	13.37
Tobacco consumption—% of smokers	29%
Tobacco consumption—cigarettes per day	14.6
Cannabis prevalence all adults 15–64	5.4
Cannabis prevalence young adults 15–34	13.5
Cannabis prevalence youth 15–24	18.9
Heroin prevalence [lower/higher]	2.81/4.7
FCTC ratification year	2004
Party to the 1961 Single Convention	1961

Annex 11: (continued) Denmark—model 3

Party to the 1961 Single Convention as amended in 1972	1975
Ratification of 1971 Convention on Psychotropic Substances	1971
Party to the 1988 Convention	1988
National public spending on drug-related activities—% of GDP	n.a.

Strategy

Responsible ministry for drug and addictions policies	Ministry of Health
The drug classification of the country determines the final penalties	Yes
Penalties for possessing drugs are higher than the EU recommendations	Yes
Penalties for trafficking drugs are higher than the EU recommendations	Yes
This country decriminalizes drug possession	No
Injection rooms—proxy for harm reduction	No
Alcohol policy scale	68/133
Alcohol price	135/234
Adopted written national policy on alcohol	Yes
Tobacco control scale	46/100
Specific national government objectives in tobacco control	Yes
Public health is included in the national strategy	No
Well-being is included in the national strategy	No
The country has EMCDDA best practices	1
Priority in the national strategy	Prevention

Structure

Ad hoc organization	No
Tackles legal and illicit substances together	No
Number of ministries involved	7/20
The country devolves policy-making to decentralized structures	Yes
The country devolves implementation to decentralized structures	Yes
Non-profit organization in the decision-making	No
Private organization in the implementation	No
Addiction is a priority in the national strategy	No

Data source: see Annex 5: Variables for factors construct and their definitions.

Annex 12: Estonia—model 4

State factors

Year of entry into the EU	2004
OECD Better Life Initiative	4/10
OECD material living conditions	2.53/10
OECD quality of life	5.47/10
Status Index	n.a.
Management Index	n.a.
Majority religion	Protestantism
Traditional vs rational values [–2 to 2]	1.27
Survival vs self-expression values [–2 to 2]	–1.19
Political structure	Unitary
Corruption Perception Index	6.4/10
Population	0.26%
GDP per capita	67
Income level	11,900
Unemployment rate	12.5%
Unemployment rate (youth)	22.3%
At risk poverty rate after social transfers	15.8%
GINI Index	31.9
Human Development Index	0.8

Policy factors

Location regarding trafficking	Transhipment and destination point
Main drug trafficked	n.a.
Alcohol consumption—recorded	13.8
Alcohol consumption—unrecorded	15.57
Tobacco consumption—% of smokers	33.3%
Tobacco consumption—cigarettes per day	n.a.
Cannabis prevalence all adults 15–64	6
Cannabis prevalence young adults 15–34	13.6
Cannabis prevalence youth 15–24	19.4
Heroin prevalence [lower/higher]	n.a.
FCTC ratification year	2005
Party to the 1961 Single Convention	–
Party to the 1961 Single Convention as amended in 1972	1996

Annex 12: (continued) Estonia—model 4

Ratification of 1971 Convention on Psychotropic Substances	1996
Party to the 1988 Convention	2000
National public spending on drug-related activities—% of GDP	0.01%

Strategy

Responsible ministry for drug and addictions policies	Ministry of Social Affairs
The drug classification of the country determines the final penalties	No
Penalties for possessing drugs are higher than the EU recommendations	Yes
Penalties for trafficking drugs are higher than the EU recommendations	Yes
This country decriminalizes drug possession	Yes
Injection rooms—proxy for harm reduction	No
Alcohol policy scale	80/133
Alcohol price	106/234
Adopted written national policy on alcohol	No
Tobacco control scale	43/100
Specific national government objectives in tobacco control	Yes
Public health is included in the national strategy	No
Well-being is included in the national strategy	No
The country has EMCDDA best practices	No
Priority in the national strategy	Prevention

Structure

Ad hoc organization	Yes
Tackles legal and illicit substances together	Yes
Number of ministries involved	4/13
The country devolves policy-making to decentralized structures	No
The country devolves implementation to decentralized structures	No
Non-profit organization in the decision-making	No
Private organization in the implementation	No
Addiction is a priority in the national strategy	No
Year of the first law on illicit substances	1997

Data source: see Annex 5: Variables for factors construct and their definitions.

Annex 13: Finland—model 2

State factors

Year of entry into the EU	1995
OECD Better Life Initiative	6.87/10
OECD material living conditions	5.53/10
OECD quality of life	8.21/10
Status Index	8.52/10
Management Index	7.79/10
Majority religion	Protestantism
Traditional vs rational values [−2 to 2]	0.82
Survival vs self-expression values [−2 to 2]	1.12
Political structure	Unitary
Corruption Perception Index	9.4
Population	1.06
GDP per capita	116
Income level	35,200
Unemployment rate	7.8
Unemployment rate (youth)	20.1
At risk poverty rate after social transfers	13.1
GINI Index	25.8
Human Development Index	0.9

Policy factors

Location regarding trafficking	Transit and final destination
Main drug trafficked	n.a.
Alcohol consumption—recorded	9.7
Alcohol consumption—unrecorded	12.52
Tobacco consumption—% of smokers	21%
Tobacco consumption—cigarettes per day	12.8
Cannabis prevalence all adults 15–64	3.6
Cannabis prevalence young adults 15–34	8
Cannabis prevalence youth 15–24	9.1
Heroin prevalence [lower/higher]	4.3/5.7
FCTC ratification year	2005
Party to the 1961 Single Convention	1961

Annex 13: (continued) Finland—model 2

Party to the 1961 Single Convention as amended in 1972	1973
Ratification of 1971 Convention on Psychotropic Substances	1971
Party to the 1988 Convention	1989
National public spending on drug-related activities—% of GDP	0.07%

Strategy

Responsible ministry for drug and addictions policies	Ministry of Health
The drug classification of the country determines the final penalties	No
Penalties for possessing drugs are higher than the EU recommendations	No
Penalties for trafficking drugs are higher than the EU recommendations	No
This country decriminalizes drug possession	Yes
Injection rooms—proxy for harm reduction	No
Alcohol policy scale	112/133
Alcohol price	170/234
Adopted written national policy on alcohol	Yes
Tobacco control scale	52
Specific national government objectives in tobacco control	Yes
Public health is included in the national strategy	No
Well-being is included in the national strategy	No
The country has EMCDDA best practices	1
Priority in the national strategy	Prevention

Structure

Ad hoc organization	Yes
Tackles legal and illicit substances together	No
Number of ministries involved	7/11
The country devolves policy-making to decentralized structures	Yes
The country devolves implementation to decentralized structures	Yes
Non-profit organization in the decision-making	No
Private organization in the implementation	No
Addiction is a priority in the national strategy	No
Year of the first law on illicit substances	1994

Data source: see Annex 5: Variables for factors construct and their definitions.

Annex 14: France—model 2

State factors

Year of entry into the EU	1952
OECD Better Life Initiative	6.54
OECD material living conditions	6.06
OECD quality of life	7.03
Status Index	8.52
Management Index	7.79
Majority religion	Catholicism
Traditional vs rational values [–2 to 2]	0.63
Survival vs self-expression values [–2 to 2]	1.13
Political structure	Unitary
Corruption Perception Index	6.8/10
Population	12.8%
GDP per capita	107
Income level	30,600
Unemployment rate	9.7
Unemployment rate (youth)	22.9
At risk poverty rate after social transfers	13.3
GINI Index	30.8
Human Development Index	0.9

Policy factors

Location regarding trafficking	Transit and final destination
Main drug trafficked	Cannabis
Alcohol consumption—recorded	13.3
Alcohol consumption—unrecorded	13.65
Tobacco consumption—% of smokers	26.1%
Tobacco consumption—cigarettes per day	12.2
Cannabis prevalence all adults 15–64	8.6
Cannabis prevalence young adults 15–34	16.7
Cannabis prevalence youth 15–24	21.7
Heroin prevalence [lower/higher]	n.a.
FCTC ratification year	2004
Party to the 1961 Single Convention	1969

Annex 14: (continued) France—model 2

Party to the 1961 Single Convention as amended in 1972	1975
Ratification of 1971 Convention on Psychotropic Substances	1971
Party to the 1988 Convention	1989
National public spending on drug-related activities—% of GDP	0.1%

Strategy

Responsible ministry for drug and addictions policies	Ministry of Health
The drug classification of the country determines the final penalties	No
Penalties for possessing drugs are higher than the EU recommendations	No
Penalties for trafficking drugs are higher than the EU recommendations	No
This country decriminalizes drug possession	No
Injection rooms—proxy for harm reduction	No
Alcohol policy scale	92/133
Alcohol price	95/234
Adopted written national policy on alcohol	No
Tobacco control scale	55/100
Specific national government objectives in tobacco control	Yes
Public health is included in the national strategy	No
Well-being is included in the national strategy	No
The country has EMCDDA best practices	1
Priority in the national strategy	Prevention

Structure

Ad hoc organization	Yes
Tackles legal and illicit substances together	Yes
Number of ministries involved	7/15
The country devolves policy-making to decentralized structures	No
The country devolves implementation to decentralized structures	Yes
Non-profit organization in the decision-making	No
Private organization in the implementation	No
Addiction is a priority in the national strategy	No
Year of the first law on illicit substances	1970

Data source: see Annex 5: Variables for factors construct and their definitions.

Annex 15: Germany—model 1

State factors	
Year of entry into the EU	1952
OECD Better Life Initiative	6.85/10
OECD material living conditions	6.2/10
OECD quality of life	7.51/10
Status Index	7.77/10
Management Index	6.84/10
Majority religion	Protestantism and Catholicism
Traditional vs rational values [–2 to 2]	1.17
Survival vs self-expression values [–2 to 2]	0.44
Political structure	Federal
Corruption Perception Index	7.9
Population	16.08%
GDP per capita	120
Income level	31,700€/year
Unemployment rate	5.9%
nemployment rate (youth)	8.6%
At risk poverty rate after social transfers	15.6%
GINI Index	29
Human Development Index	0.9
Policy factors	
Location regarding trafficking	Traffic and final destination.
Main drug trafficked	Synthetic drugs and cannabis
Alcohol consumption—recorded	11.8
Alcohol consumption—unrecorded	12.81
Tobacco consumption—% of smokers	25%
Tobacco consumption—cigarettes per day	14.7
Cannabis prevalence all adults 15–64	4.8
Cannabis prevalence young adults 15–34	11.1
Cannabis prevalence youth 15–24	15.1
Heroin prevalence [lower/higher]	2.27/3.03
FCTC ratification year	2004

Annex 15: (continued) Germany—model 1

Party to the 1961 Single Convention	1961
Party to the 1961 Single Convention as amended in 1972	1975
Ratification of 1971 Convention on Psychotropic Substances	1971
Party to the 1988 Convention	1989
National public spending on drug-related activities—% of GDP	0.23–0.26%

Strategy

Responsible ministry for drug and addictions policies	Ministry of Health
The drug classification of the country determines the final penalties	No
Penalties for possessing drugs are higher than the EU recommendations	Yes
Penalties for trafficking drugs are higher than the EU recommendations	Yes
This country decriminalizes drug possession	Yes
Injection rooms—proxy for harm reduction	Yes
Alcohol policy scale	45/133
Alcohol price	91/234
Adopted written national policy on alcohol	Yes
Tobacco control scale	37/100
Specific national government objectives in tobacco control	Yes
Public health is included in the national strategy	No
Well-being is included in the national strategy	No
The country has EMCDDA best practices	1, 2, & 3
Priority in the national strategy	Prevention

Structure

Ad hoc organization	Yes
Tackles legal and illicit substances together	Yes
Number of ministries involved	7/15
The country devolves policy-making to decentralized structures	Yes
The country devolves implementation to decentralized structures	Yes
Non-profit organization in the decision-making	Yes
Private organization in the implementation	No
Addiction is a priority in the national strategy	Yes
Year of the first law on illicit substances	1929

Data source: see Annex 5: Variables for factors construct and their definitions.

Annex 16: Greece—model 4

State factors	
Year of entry into the EU	1981
OECD Better Life Initiative	4.9/10
OECD material living conditions	4.1/10
OECD quality of life	5.7/10
Status Index	5.12/10
Management Index	4.54/10
Majority religion	Orthodoxy
Traditional vs rational values [–2 to 2]	0.77
Survival vs self-expression values [–2 to 2]	0.55
Political structure	Unitary
Corruption Perception Index	3.5/10
Population	2.23%
GDP per capita	82
Income level	18,500€/year
Unemployment rate	17.7%
Unemployment rate (youth)	44.4%
At risk poverty rate after social transfers	20.1%
GINI Index	33.6
Human Development Index	0.9

Policy factors	
Location regarding trafficking	Gateway of Balkan route
Main drug trafficked	Heroin
Alcohol consumption—recorded	9
Alcohol consumption—unrecorded	10.75
Tobacco consumption—% of smokers	27.6%
Tobacco consumption—cigarettes per day	21.4
Cannabis prevalence all adults 15–64	1.7
Cannabis prevalence young adults 15–34	3.2
Cannabis prevalence youth 15–24	1.19
Heroin prevalence [lower/higher]	1.69/–
FCTC ratification year	2006
Party to the 1961 Single Convention	–

Annex 16: (continued) Greece—model 4

Party to the 1961 Single Convention as amended in 1972	–
Ratification of 1971 Convention on Psychotropic Substances	–
Party to the 1988 Convention	–
National public spending on drug-related activities—% of GDP	0.05%

Strategy

Responsible ministry for drug and addictions policies	Ministry of Health
The drug classification of the country determines the final penalties	No
Penalties for possessing drugs are higher than the EU recommendations	No
Penalties for trafficking drugs are higher than the EU recommendations	Yes
This country decriminalizes drug possession	No
Injection rooms—proxy for harm reduction	No
Alcohol policy scale	55/133
Alcohol price	105/234
Adopted written national policy on alcohol	No
Tobacco control scale	32/100
Specific national government objectives in tobacco control	No
Public health is included in the national strategy	No
Well-being is included in the national strategy	No
The country has EMCDDA best practices	1 & 2
Priority in the national strategy	National coordination

Structure

Ad hoc organization	Yes
Tackles legal and illicit substances together	Yes
Number of ministries involved	9/18
The country devolves policy-making to decentralized structures	No
The country devolves implementation to decentralized structures	No
Non-profit organization in the decision-making	No
Private organization in the implementation	No
Addiction is a priority in the national strategy	No
Year of the first law on illicit substances	1987

Data source: see Annex 5: Variables for factors construct and their definitions.

Annex 17: Hungary—model 4

State factors	
Year of entry into the EU	2004
OECD Better Life Initiative	4.31/10
OECD material living conditions	2.9/10
OECD quality of life	5.72
Status Index	5.94/10
Management Index	5.71/10
Majority religion	Catholicism
Traditional vs rational values [−2 to 2]	0.4
Survival vs self-expression values [−2 to 2]	−1.22
Political structure	Unitary
Corruption Perception Index	4.7/10
Population	1.96%
GDP per capita	66
Income level	10,000€/year
Unemployment rate	26.1%
Unemployment rate (youth)	4.3%
At risk poverty rate after social transfers	12.3%
GINI Index	26.9
Human Development Index	0.8
Policy factors	
Location regarding trafficking	Heroin and cannabis
Main drug trafficked	Transhipment point for heroin and cannabis
Alcohol consumption—recorded	12.3
Alcohol consumption—unrecorded	16.27
Tobacco consumption—% of smokers	38%
Tobacco consumption—cigarettes per day	16.3
Cannabis prevalence all adults 15–64	2.3
Cannabis prevalence young adults 15–34	5.7
Cannabis prevalence youth 15–24	10.1
Heroin prevalence [lower/higher]	n.a.
FCTC ratification year	n.a.
Party to the 1961 Single Convention	2004

Annex 17: (continued) Hungary—model 4

Party to the 1961 Single Convention as amended in 1972	1961
Ratification of 1971 Convention on Psychotropic Substances	1987
Party to the 1988 Convention	1971
National public spending on drug-related activities—% of GDP	0.04%

Strategy

Responsible ministry for drug and addictions policies	Ministry of Social Affairs and Labour
The drug classification of the country determines the final penalties	No
Penalties for possessing drugs are higher than the EU recommendations	No
Penalties for trafficking drugs are higher than the EU recommendations	Yes
This country decriminalizes drug possession	No
Injection rooms—proxy for harm reduction	No
Alcohol policy scale	60/133
Alcohol price	84/234
Adopted written national policy on alcohol	No
Tobacco control scale	34/100
Specific national government objectives in tobacco control	Yes
Public health is included in the national strategy	No
Well-being is included in the national strategy	No
The country has EMCDDA best practices	1
Priority in the national strategy	Prevention

Structure

Ad hoc organization	Yes
Tackles legal and illicit substances together	Yes
Number of ministries involved	8/8
The country devolves policy-making to decentralized structures	No
The country devolves implementation to decentralized structures	No
Non-profit organization in the decision-making	Yes
Private organization in the implementation	No
Addiction is a priority in the national strategy	No
Year of the first law on illicit substances	1930

Data source: see Annex 5: Variables for factors construct and their definitions.

Annex 18: Ireland—model 2

State factors	
Year of entry into the EU	1973
OECD Better Life Initiative	6.84/10
OECD material living conditions	5.86/10
OECD quality of life	7.83/10
Status Index	7.37/10
Management Index	6.33/10
Majority religion	Catholicism
Traditional vs rational values [−2 to 2]	−0.91
Survival vs self-expression values [−2 to 2]	1.18
Political structure	Unitary
Corruption Perception Index	8/10
Population	0.88%
GDP per capita	127
Income level	35,400€/year
Unemployment rate	14.4
Unemployment rate (youth)	29.4
At risk poverty rate after social transfers	16.1%
GINI Index	33.2
Human Development Index	0.9
Policy factors	
Location regarding trafficking	Transhipment for cannabis and synthetic drugs.
Main drug trafficked	Cannabis
Alcohol consumption—recorded	13.4
Alcohol consumption—unrecorded	14.41
Tobacco consumption—% of smokers	31%
Tobacco consumption—cigarettes per day	16
Cannabis prevalence all adults 15–64	6.3
Cannabis prevalence young adults 15–34	10.4
Cannabis prevalence youth 15–24	13.1
Heroin prevalence [lower/higher]	2/3.37
FCTC ratification year	2005
Party to the 1961 Single Convention	1980

Annex 18: (continued) Ireland—model 2

Party to the 1961 Single Convention as amended in 1972	1980
Ratification of 1971 Convention on Psychotropic Substances	1992
Party to the 1988 Convention	1989
National public spending on drug-related activities—% of GDP	0.17%

Strategy

Responsible ministry for drug and addictions policies	Ministry of Health
The drug classification of the country determines the final penalties	Yes
Penalties for possessing drugs are higher than the EU recommendations	Yes
Penalties for trafficking drugs are higher than the EU recommendations	Yes
This country decriminalizes drug possession	Yes
Injection rooms—proxy for harm reduction	No
Alcohol policy scale	83/133
Alcohol price	167/234
Adopted written national policy on alcohol	Yes
Tobacco control scale	69/100
Specific national government objectives in tobacco control	Yes
Public health is included in the national strategy	No
Well-being is included in the national strategy	No
The country has EMCDDA best practices	1 & 2
Priority in the national strategy	Supply reduction

Structure

Ad hoc organization	Yes
Tackles legal and illicit substances together	Yes
Number of ministries involved	6/14
The country devolves policy-making to decentralized structures	No
The country devolves implementation to decentralized structures	Yes
Non-profit organization in the decision-making	Yes
Private organization in the implementation	No
Addiction is a priority in the national strategy	No
Year of the first law on illicit substances	1977

Data source: see Annex 5: Variables for factors construct and their definitions.

Annex 19: Italy—model 1

State factors	
Year of entry into the EU	1952
OECD Better Life Initiative	5.94/10
OECD material living conditions	5.46/10
OECD quality of life	6.43/10
Status Index	5.7/10
Management Index	5.62/10
Majority religion	Catholicism
Traditional vs rational values [–2 to 2]	0.13
Survival vs self-expression values [–2 to 2]	0.6
Political structure	Regionalized
Corruption Perception Index	3.9
Population	11.92%
GDP per capita	101
Income level	26,000€/year
Unemployment rate	8.4%
Unemployment rate (youth)	29.1%
At risk poverty rate after social transfers	18.2%
GINI Index	31.2
Human Development Index	0.9

Policy factors	
Location regarding trafficking	Entry point and traffic
Main drug trafficked	Cannabis
Alcohol consumption—recorded	8.3
Alcohol consumption—unrecorded	10.68
Tobacco consumption—% of smokers	24.5
Tobacco consumption—cigarettes per day	13
Cannabis prevalence all adults 15–64	14.3
Cannabis prevalence young adults 15–34	20.3
Cannabis prevalence youth 15–24	22.3
Heroin prevalence [lower/higher]	9.7/10.2
FCTC ratification year	2008
Party to the 1961 Single Convention	1961
Party to the 1961 Single Convention as amended in 1972	1975

Annex 19: (continued) Italy—model 1

Ratification of 1971 Convention on Psychotropic Substances	1981
Party to the 1988 Convention	1988
National public spending on drug-related activities—% of GDP	0.25%

Strategy

Responsible ministry for drug and addictions policies	Anti-drug department—Council of Ministers
The drug classification of the country determines the final penalties	Yes
Penalties for possessing drugs are higher than the EU recommendations	No
Penalties for trafficking drugs are higher than the EU recommendations	Yes
This country decriminalizes drug possession	Yes
Injection rooms—proxy for harm reduction	No
Alcohol policy scale	51/133
Alcohol price	113/234
Adopted written national policy on alcohol	Yes
Tobacco control scale	47/100
Specific national government objectives in tobacco control	Yes
Public health is included in the national strategy	No
Well-being is included in the national strategy	No
The country has EMCDDA best practices	1, 2, & 3
Priority in the national strategy	Prevention

Structure

Ad hoc organization	Yes
Tackles legal and illicit substances together	No
Number of ministries involved	14/14
The country devolves policy-making to decentralized structures	Yes
The country devolves implementation to decentralized structures	Yes
Non-profit organization in the decision-making	No
Private organization in the implementation	No
Addiction is a priority in the national strategy	No
Year of the first law on illicit substances	1975

Data source: see Annex 5: Variables for factors construct and their definitions.

Annex 20: Latvia—model 4

State factors

Year of entry into the EU	2004
OECD Better Life Initiative	n.a.
OECD material living conditions	n.a.
OECD quality of life	n.a.
Status Index	n.a.
Management Index	n.a.
Majority religion	Protestantism and Catholicism
Traditional vs rational values [−2 to 2]	0.72
Survival vs self-expression values [−2 to 2]	−1.27
Political structure	Unitary
Corruption Perception Index	4.2
Population	0.44%
GDP per capita	58
Income level	9,800€/year
Unemployment rate	15.4
Unemployment rate (youth)	29.1
At risk poverty rate after social transfers	21.3%
GINI Index	35.2
Human Development Index	0.8

Policy factors

Location regarding trafficking	Transhipment and destination point
Main drug trafficked	n.a.
Alcohol consumption—recorded	9.5
Alcohol consumption—unrecorded	12.5
Tobacco consumption—% of smokers	32.7%
Tobacco consumption—cigarettes per day	13.1
Cannabis prevalence all adults 15–64	4.9
Cannabis prevalence young adults 15–34	9.7
Cannabis prevalence youth 15–24	12.9
Heroin prevalence [lower/higher]	3.1/6.2
FCTC ratification year	2005
Party to the 1961 Single Convention	1993

Annex 20: (continued) Latvia—model 4

Party to the 1961 Single Convention as amended in 1972	1993
Ratification of 1971 Convention on Psychotropic Substances	1993
Party to the 1988 Convention	1994
National public spending on drug-related activities—% of GDP	0.01%

Strategy

Responsible ministry for drug and addictions policies	Ministry of Interior
The drug classification of the country determines the final penalties	No
Penalties for possessing drugs are higher than the EU recommendations	No
Penalties for trafficking drugs are higher than the EU recommendations	Yes
This country decriminalizes drug possession	Yes
Injection rooms—proxy for harm reduction	No
Alcohol policy scale	78/133
Alcohol price	118/234
Adopted written national policy on alcohol	Yes
Tobacco control scale	44/100
Specific national government objectives in tobacco control	Yes
Public health is included in the national strategy	No
Well-being is included in the national strategy	No
The country has EMCDDA best practices	1
Priority in the national strategy	Prevention

Structure

Ad hoc organization	Yes
Tackles legal and illicit substances together	No
Number of ministries involved	7/13
The country devolves policy-making to decentralized structures	No
The country devolves implementation to decentralized structures	No
Non-profit organization in the decision-making	No
Private organization in the implementation	No
Addiction is a priority in the national strategy	No
Year of the first law on illicit substances	1993

Data source: see Annex 5: Variables for factors construct and their definitions.

Annex 21: Lithuania—model 4

State factors	
Year of entry into the EU	2004
OECD Better Life Initiative	n.a.
OECD material living conditions	n.a.
OECD quality of life	n.a.
Status Index	n.a.
Management Index	n.a.
Majority religion	Catholicism
Traditional vs rational values [−2 to 2]	0.98
Survival vs self-expression values [−2 to 2]	−1
Political structure	Unitary
Corruption Perception Index	4.8
Population	0.64%
GDP per capita	62
Income level	10,200€/year
Unemployment rate	15.4%
Unemployment rate (youth)	32.9%
At risk poverty rate after social transfers	20.2
GINI Index	32.9
Human Development Index	0.8
Policy factors	
Location regarding trafficking	Transhipment and destination point.
Main drug trafficked	n.a.
Alcohol consumption—recorded	12
Alcohol consumption—unrecorded	15.03
Tobacco consumption—% of smokers	30%
Tobacco consumption—cigarettes per day	12.6
Cannabis prevalence all adults 15–64	5.6
Cannabis prevalence young adults 15–34	9.9
Cannabis prevalence youth 15–24	12.8
Heroin prevalence [lower/higher]	n.a.
FCTC ratification year	2004
Party to the 1961 Single Convention	1994
Party to the 1961 Single Convention as amended in 1972	1994

Annex 21: (continued) Lithuania—model 4

Ratification of 1971 Convention on Psychotropic Substances	1994
Party to the 1988 Convention	1998
National public spending on drug-related activities—% of GDP	0.02%

Strategy

Responsible ministry for drug and addictions policies	Prime minister
The drug classification of the country determines the final penalties	No
Penalties for possessing drugs are higher than the EU recommendations	Yes
Penalties for trafficking drugs are higher than the EU recommendations	Yes
This country decriminalizes drug possession	Yes
Injection rooms—proxy for harm reduction	No
Alcohol policy scale	82/133
Alcohol price	99/234
Adopted written national policy on alcohol	Yes
Tobacco control scale	41/100
Specific national government objectives in tobacco control	Yes
Public health is included in the national strategy	Yes
Well-being is included in the national strategy	No
The country has EMCDDA best practices	1
Priority in the national strategy	Demand reduction

Structure

Ad hoc organization	Yes
Tackles legal and illicit substances together	No
Number of ministries involved	13/14
The country devolves policy-making to decentralized structures	No
The country devolves implementation to decentralized structures	No
Non-profit organization in the decision-making	No
Private organization in the implementation	No
Addiction is a priority in the national strategy	Yes
Year of the first law on illicit substances	1998

Data source: see Annex 5: Variables for factors construct and their definitions.

Annex 22: Luxembourg—model 1

State factors

Year of entry into the EU	1952
OECD Better Life Initiative	7.5/10
OECD material living conditions	7.56/10
OECD quality of life	7.45/10
Status Index	7.60/10
Management Index	7.05/10
Majority religion	Catholicism
Traditional vs rational values [–2 to 2]	0.42
Survival vs self-expression values [–2 to 2]	1.13
Political structure	Unitary
Corruption Perception Index	8.5
Population	0.1%
GDP per capita	274
Income level	82,100€/year
Unemployment rate	4.8%
Unemployment rate (youth)	15.6%
At risk poverty rate after social transfers	14.5%
GINI Index	27.2
Human Development Index	0.9

Policy factors

Location regarding trafficking	Traffic and final destination
Main drug trafficked	Cannabis and synthetic substances
Alcohol consumption—recorded	12
Alcohol consumption—unrecorded	13.01
Tobacco consumption—% of smokers	25%
Tobacco consumption—cigarettes per day	17.2
Cannabis prevalence all adults 15–64	n.a.
Cannabis prevalence young adults 15–34	n.a.
Cannabis prevalence youth 15–24	n.a.
Heroin prevalence [lower/higher]	3.9/6
FCTC ratification year	2005

Annex 22: (continued) Luxembourg—model 1

Party to the 1961 Single Convention	1961
Party to the 1961 Single Convention as amended in 1972	1987
Ratification of 1971 Convention on Psychotropic Substances	1993
Party to the 1988 Convention	1989
National public spending on drug-related activities—% of GDP	0.1%

Strategy

Responsible ministry for drug and addictions policies	Ministry of Health
The drug classification of the country determines the final penalties	Yes
Penalties for possessing drugs are higher than the EU recommendations	No
Penalties for trafficking drugs are higher than the EU recommendations	Yes
This country decriminalizes drug possession	Yes
Injection rooms—proxy for harm reduction	Yes
Alcohol policy scale	387,133
Alcohol price	96/234
Adopted written national policy on alcohol	No
Tobacco control scale	33/100
Specific national government objectives in tobacco control	No
Public health is included in the national strategy	Yes
Well-being is included in the national strategy	No
The country has EMCDDA best practices	1
Priority in the national strategy	Prevention

Structure

Ad hoc organization	Yes
Tackles legal and illicit substances together	Yes
Number of ministries involved	10/18
The country devolves policy-making to decentralized structures	No
The country devolves implementation to decentralized structures	No
Non-profit organization in the decision-making	Yes
Private organization in the implementation	No
Addiction is a priority in the national strategy	No
Year of the first law on illicit substances	1973

Data source: see Annex 5: Variables for factors construct and their definitions.

Annex 23: Malta—model 4

State factors	
Year of entry into the EU	2004
OECD Better Life Initiative	n.a.
OECD material living conditions	n.a.
OECD quality of life	n.a.
Status Index	n.a.
Management Index	n.a.
Majority religion	Catholicism
Traditional vs rational values [–2 to 2]	n.a.
Survival vs self-expression values [–2 to 2]	n.a.
Political structure	Unitary
Corruption Perception Index	5.6/10
Population	0.08%
GDP per capita	83
Income level	15,500€/year
Unemployment rate	6.5
Unemployment rate (youth)	13.7
At risk poverty rate after social transfers	15%
GINI Index	27.4
Human Development Index	0.8
Policy factors	
Location regarding trafficking	n.a.
Main drug trafficked	n.a.
Alcohol consumption—recorded	3.9
Alcohol consumption—unrecorded	4.3
Tobacco consumption—% of smokers	25.7%
Tobacco consumption—cigarettes per day	16.3
Cannabis prevalence all adults 15–64	0.8
Cannabis prevalence young adults 15–34	1.9
Cannabis prevalence youth 15–24	n.a.
Heroin prevalence [lower/higher]	5.5/6
FCTC ratification year	2003
Party to the 1961 Single Convention	1990
Party to the 1961 Single Convention as amended in 1972	1990

Annex 23: (continued) Malta—model 4

Ratification of 1971 Convention on Psychotropic Substances	1990
Party to the 1988 Convention	1996
National public spending on drug-related activities—% of GDP	n.a.

Strategy

Responsible ministry for drug and addictions policies	Ministry of Justice, Dialogue and the Family
The drug classification of the country determines the final penalties	No
Penalties for possessing drugs are higher than the EU recommendations	Yes
Penalties for trafficking drugs are higher than the EU recommendations	Yes
This country decriminalizes drug possession	No
Injection rooms—proxy for harm reduction	No
Alcohol policy scale	39/133
Alcohol price	98/100
Adopted written national policy on alcohol	No
Tobacco control scale	52/100
Specific national government objectives in tobacco control	No
Public health is included in the national strategy	Yes
Well-being is included in the national strategy	Yes
The country has EMCDDA best practices	No
Priority in the national strategy	National coordination

Structure

Ad hoc organization	Yes
Tackles legal and illicit substances together	No
Number of ministries involved	7/14
The country devolves policy-making to decentralized structures	No
The country devolves implementation to decentralized structures	No
Non-profit organization in the decision-making	No
Private organization in the implementation	No
Addiction is a priority in the national strategy	No
Year of the first law on illicit substances	1901

Data source: see Annex 5: Variables for factors construct and their definitions.

Annex 24: The Netherlands—model 1

State factors	
Year of entry into the EU	1952
OECD Better Life Initiative	7.55/10
OECD material living conditions	7.26/10
OECD quality of life	7.85/10
Status Index	7.63/10
Management Index	6.84/10
Majority religion	Protestantism and Catholicism
Traditional vs rational values [–2 to 2]	0.71
Survival vs self-expression values [–2 to 2]	1.39
Political structure	Regionalized
Corruption Perception Index	8.8/10
Population	3,28%
GDP per capita	131
Income level	36,100€
Unemployment rate	4.4%
Unemployment rate (youth)	7,6
At risk poverty rate after social transfers	10,3%
GINI Index	25,8
Human Development Index	0.9
Policy factors	
Location regarding trafficking	Production and traffic
Main drug trafficked	Cannabis
Alcohol consumption—recorded	9.6
Alcohol consumption—unrecorded	10.06
Tobacco consumption—% of smokers	24
Tobacco consumption—cigarettes per day	14.2
Cannabis prevalence all adults 15–64	5.4
Cannabis prevalence young adults 15–34	9.5
Cannabis prevalence youth 15–24	11.4
Heroin prevalence [lower/higher]	0.2/0.4
FCTC ratification year	2005
Party to the 1961 Single Convention	1961
Party to the 1961 Single Convention as amended in 1972	1987

Annex 24: (continued) The Netherlands—model 1

Ratification of 1971 Convention on Psychotropic Substances	1993
Party to the 1988 Convention	1989
National public spending on drug-related activities—% of GDP	0.5%

Strategy

Responsible ministry for drug and addictions policies	Ministry of Health
The drug classification of the country determines the final penalties	Yes
Penalties for possessing drugs are higher than the EU recommendations	No
Penalties for trafficking drugs are higher than the EU recommendations	Yes
This country decriminalizes drug possession	Yes
Injection rooms—proxy for harm reduction	Yes
Alcohol policy scale	63/133
Alcohol price	99/234
Adopted written national policy on alcohol	Yes
Tobacco control scale	46/100
Specific national government objectives in tobacco control	Yes
Public health is included in the national strategy	No
Well-being is included in the national strategy	No
The country has EMCDDA best practices	1, 2, & 3
Priority in the national strategy	Prevention

Structure

Ad hoc organization	No
Tackles legal and illicit substances together	No
Number of ministries involved	5/11
The country devolves policy-making to decentralized structures	Yes
The country devolves implementation to decentralized structures	Yes
Non-profit organization in the decision-making	No
Private organization in the implementation	No
Addiction is a priority in the national strategy	No
Year of the first law on illicit substances	1919

Data source: see Annex 5: Variables for factors construct and their definitions.

Annex 25: Norway—model 2

State factors	
Year of entry into the EU	Not an EU member
OECD Better Life Initiative	7.53/10
OECD material living conditions	6.73/10
OECD quality of life	8.33/10
Status Index	8.64/10
Management Index	8.2/10
Majority religion	Protestantism
Traditional vs rational values [–2 to 2]	1.39
Survival vs self-expression values [–2 to 2]	2.17
Political structure	Unitary
Corruption Perception Index	9/10
Population	0.97%
GDP per capita	189
Income level	70,500€/year
Unemployment rate	3.3%
Unemployment rate (youth)	8.9%
At risk poverty rate after social transfers	11.2
GINI Index	22.9
Human Development Index	0.9
Policy factors	
Location regarding trafficking	Final destination
Main drug trafficked	Cannabis
Alcohol consumption—recorded	6.2
Alcohol consumption—unrecorded	7.81
Tobacco consumption—% of smokers	n.a.
Tobacco consumption—cigarettes per day	n.a.
Cannabis prevalence all adults 15–64	3.8
Cannabis prevalence young adults 15–34	7
Cannabis prevalence youth 15–24	8.4
Heroin prevalence [lower/higher]	2.8/3.9
FCTC ratification year	2003
Party to the 1961 Single Convention	1961
Party to the 1961 Single Convention as amended in 1972	1973

Annex 25: (continued) Norway—model 2

Ratification of 1971 Convention on Psychotropic Substances	1975
Party to the 1988 Convention	1988
National public spending on drug-related activities—% of GDP	n.a.

Strategy

Responsible ministry for drug and addictions policies	Ministry of Health and Care Services
The drug classification of the country determines the final penalties	No
Penalties for possessing drugs are higher than the EU recommendations	Yes
Penalties for trafficking drugs are higher than the EU recommendations	Yes
This country decriminalizes drug possession	No
Injection rooms—proxy for harm reduction	Yes
Alcohol policy scale	133/133
Alcohol price	234/234
Adopted written national policy on alcohol	Yes
Tobacco control scale	62/100
Specific national government objectives in tobacco control	Yes
Public health is included in the national strategy	Yes
Well-being is included in the national strategy	No
The country has EMCDDA best practices	1 & 2
Priority in the national strategy	Treatment and rehabilitation

Structure

Ad hoc organization	Yes
Tackles legal and illicit substances together	Yes
Number of ministries involved	9/17
The country devolves policy-making to decentralized structures	No
The country devolves implementation to decentralized structures	Yes
Non-profit organization in the decision-making	No
Private organization in the implementation	No
Addiction is a priority in the national strategy	No
Year of the first law on illicit substances	1902

Data source: see Annex 5: Variables for factors construct and their definitions.

Annex 26: Poland—model 3

State factors	
Year of entry into the EU	2004
OECD Better Life Initiative	4.7/10
OECD material living conditions	3.33/10
OECD quality of life	6.08/10
Status Index	6.33/10
Management Index	5.79/10
Majority religion	Catholicism
Traditional vs rational values [−2 to 2]	−0.78
Survival vs self-expression values [−2 to 2]	−0.14
Political structure	Unitary
Corruption Perception Index	6/10
Population	7.51%
GDP per capita	65
Income level	9,300€/year
Unemployment rate	9.7%
Unemployment rate (youth)	25.8%
At risk poverty rate after social transfers	17.6%
GINI Index	31.1
Human Development Index	0.8

Policy factors	
Location regarding trafficking	Illicit producer of synthetic substances
Main drug trafficked	Synthetic substances
Alcohol consumption—recorded	9.6
Alcohol consumption—unrecorded	13.25
Tobacco consumption—% of smokers	29.9%
Tobacco consumption—cigarettes per day	15.3
Cannabis prevalence all adults 15–64	2.7
Cannabis prevalence young adults 15–34	5.3
Cannabis prevalence youth 15–24	7.5
Heroin prevalence [lower/higher]	3.7/4.7
FCTC ratification year	2006
Party to the 1961 Single Convention	1961

Annex 26: (continued) Poland—model 3

Party to the 1961 Single Convention as amended in 1972	1993
Ratification of 1971 Convention on Psychotropic Substances	1975
Party to the 1988 Convention	1989
National public spending on drug-related activities—% of GDP	0.2%

Strategy

Responsible ministry for drug and addictions policies	Ministry of Health
The drug classification of the country determines the final penalties	No
Penalties for possessing drugs are higher than the EU recommendations	Yes
Penalties for trafficking drugs are higher than the EU recommendations	No
This country decriminalizes drug possession	No
Injection rooms—proxy for harm reduction	No
Alcohol policy scale	86/133
Alcohol price	89/234
Adopted written national policy on alcohol	Yes
Tobacco control scale	43/100
Specific national government objectives in tobacco control	Yes
Public health is included in the national strategy	No
Well-being is included in the national strategy	No
The country has EMCDDA best practices	1, 2, & 3
Priority in the national strategy	Prevention

Structure

Ad hoc organization	Yes
Tackles legal and illicit substances together	No
Number of ministries involved	8/18
The country devolves policy-making to decentralized structures	Yes
The country devolves implementation to decentralized structures	Yes
Non-profit organization in the decision-making	No
Private organization in the implementation	No
Addiction is a priority in the national strategy	No
Year of the first law on illicit substances	1985

Data source: see Annex 5: Variables for factors construct and their definitions.

Annex 27: Portugal—model 1

State factors	
Year of entry into the EU	1986
OECD Better Life Initiative	5.1/10
OECD material living conditions	4.76/10
OECD quality of life	5.45/10
Status Index	6.59/10
Management Index	5.76/10
Majority religion	Catholicism
Traditional vs rational values [–2 to 2]	–0.9
Survival vs self-expression values [–2 to 2]	0.49
Political structure	Unitary
Corruption Perception Index	6.1/10
Population	2.09%
GDP per capita	65
Income level	16,000€/year
Unemployment rate	12.9%
Unemployment rate (youth)	30.1%
At risk poverty rate after social transfers	17.9%
GINI Index	34.2
Human Development Index	0.8
Policy factors	
Location regarding trafficking	Entry point
Main drug trafficked	Cannabis and cocaine
Alcohol consumption—recorded	12.5
Alcohol consumption—unrecorded	14.55
Tobacco consumption—% of smokers	16.4%
Tobacco consumption—cigarettes per day	15.5
Cannabis prevalence all adults 15–64	3.6
Cannabis prevalence young adults 15–34	6.7
Cannabis prevalence youth 15–24	6.6
Heroin prevalence [lower/higher]	4.3/7.4
FCTC ratification year	2005
Party to the 1961 Single Convention	1961
Party to the 1961 Single Convention as amended in 1972	1979

Annex 27: (continued) Portugal—model 1

Ratification of 1971 Convention on Psychotropic Substances	1979
Party to the 1988 Convention	1989
National public spending on drug-related activities—% of GDP	0.03%

Strategy

Responsible ministry for drug and addictions policies	Ministry of Health
The drug classification of the country determines the final penalties	Yes
Penalties for possessing drugs are higher than the EU recommendations	No
Penalties for trafficking drugs are higher than the EU recommendations	Yes
This country decriminalizes drug possession	Yes
Injection rooms—proxy for harm reduction	No
Alcohol policy scale	48/133
Alcohol price	86/234
Adopted written national policy on alcohol	Yes
Tobacco control scale	43/100
Specific national government objectives in tobacco control	Yes
Public health is included in the national strategy	No
Well-being is included in the national strategy	No
The country has EMCDDA best practices	1, 2, & 3
Priority in the national strategy	National coordination

Structure

Ad hoc organization	Yes
Tackles legal and illicit substances together	No
Number of ministries involved	12/16
The country devolves policy-making to decentralized structures	No
The country devolves implementation to decentralized structures	Yes
Non-profit organization in the decision-making	Yes
Private organization in the implementation	Yes
Addiction is a priority in the national strategy	No
Year of the first law on illicit substances	1993

Data source: see Annex 5: Variables for factors construct and their definitions.

Annex 28: Romania—model 4

State factors

Year of entry into the EU	2007
OECD Better Life Initiative	n.a.
OECD material living conditions	n.a.
OECD quality of life	n.a.
Status Index	n.a.
Management Index	n.a.
Majority religion	Orthodoxy
Traditional vs rational values [–2 to 2]	–0.39
Survival vs self-expression values [–2 to 2]	–1.55
Political structure	Unitary
Corruption Perception Index	4.3/10
Population	4.21%
GDP per capita	49
Income level	5,800€/year
Unemployment rate	7.4
Unemployment rate (youth)	23.7
At risk poverty rate after social transfers	21.1%
GINI Index	33.2
Human Development Index	0.8

Policy factors

Location regarding trafficking	Transhipment point in the Balkan route
Main drug trafficked	Heroin
Alcohol consumption—recorded	11.3
Alcohol consumption—unrecorded	15.3
Tobacco consumption—% of smokers	30%
Tobacco consumption—cigarettes per day	15
Cannabis prevalence all adults 15–64	0.4
Cannabis prevalence young adults 15–34	0.9
Cannabis prevalence youth 15–24	1.5
Heroin prevalence [lower/higher]	n.a.
FCTC ratification year	2006
Party to the 1961 Single Convention	1974

Annex 28: (continued) Romania—model 4

Party to the 1961 Single Convention as amended in 1972	1974
Ratification of 1971 Convention on Psychotropic Substances	1993
Party to the 1988 Convention	1993
National public spending on drug-related activities—% of GDP	0.02–0.08%

Strategy

Responsible ministry for drug and addictions policies	Prime minister
The drug classification of the country determines the final penalties	No
Penalties for possessing drugs are higher than the EU recommendations	No
Penalties for trafficking drugs are higher than the EU recommendations	Yes
This country decriminalizes drug possession	No
Injection rooms—proxy for harm reduction	No
Alcohol policy scale	72/133
Alcohol price	70/234
Adopted written national policy on alcohol	Yes
Tobacco control scale	45/100
Specific national government objectives in tobacco control	No
Public health is included in the national strategy	No
Well-being is included in the national strategy	No
The country has EMCDDA best practices	No
Priority in the national strategy	Demand reduction

Structure

Ad hoc organization	Yes
Tackles legal and illicit substances together	No
Number of ministries involved	6/24
The country devolves policy-making to decentralized structures	No
The country devolves implementation to decentralized structures	No
Non-profit organization in the decision-making	No
Private organization in the implementation	No
Addiction is a priority in the national strategy	No
Year of the first law on illicit substances	1928

Data source: see Annex 5: Variables for factors construct and their definitions.

Annex 29: Slovakia—model 4

State factors

Year of entry into the EU	2004
OECD Better Life Initiative	4.66/10
OECD material living conditions	3.1/10
OECD quality of life	6.22/10
Status Index	5.48/10
Management Index	4.75/10
Majority religion	Catholicism
Traditional vs rational values [–2 to 2]	0.67
Survival vs self-expression values [–2 to 2]	–0.43
Political structure	Regionalized
Corruption Perception Index	6.4/10
Population	1.08%
GDP per capita	73
Income level	12,700€
Unemployment rate	13.5%
Unemployment rate (youth)	33.2%
At risk poverty rate after social transfers	12%
GINI Index	25.9
Human Development Index	0.8

Policy factors

Location regarding trafficking	Transit point for illicit substances.
Main drug trafficked	Cannabis
Alcohol consumption—recorded	10.3
Alcohol consumption—unrecorded	13.33
Tobacco consumption—% of smokers	19.2%
Tobacco consumption—cigarettes per day	13.5
Cannabis prevalence all adults 15–64	6.9
Cannabis prevalence young adults 15–34	14.7
Cannabis prevalence youth 15–24	20.4
Heroin prevalence [lower/higher]	2/3
FCTC ratification year	2004
Party to the 1961 Single Convention	1993

Annex 29: (continued) Slovakia—model 4

Party to the 1961 Single Convention as amended in 1972	1993
Ratification of 1971 Convention on Psychotropic Substances	1993
Party to the 1988 Convention	1993
National public spending on drug-related activities—% of GDP	0.05%

Strategy

Responsible ministry for drug and addictions policies	Prime minister
The drug classification of the country determines the final penalties	No
Penalties for possessing drugs are higher than the EU recommendations	No
Penalties for trafficking drugs are higher than the EU recommendations	No
This country decriminalizes drug possession	No
Injection rooms—proxy for harm reduction	No
Alcohol policy scale	62/133
Alcohol price	102/234
Adopted written national policy on alcohol	1
Tobacco control scale	41/100
Specific national government objectives in tobacco control	1
Public health is included in the national strategy	No
Well-being is included in the national strategy	No
The country has EMCDDA best practices	1 & 2
Priority in the national strategy	Demand reduction

Structure

Ad hoc organization	Yes
Tackles legal and illicit substances together	No
Number of ministries involved	14/14
The country devolves policy-making to decentralized structures	No
The country devolves implementation to decentralized structures	No
Non-profit organization in the decision-making	No
Private organization in the implementation	Yes
Addiction is a priority in the national strategy	No
Year of the first law on illicit substances	1967

Data source: see Annex 5: Variables for factors construct and their definitions.

Annex 30: Slovenia—model 3

State factors	
Year of entry into the EU	2004
OECD Better Life Initiative	5.82/10
OECD material living conditions	4.86/10
OECD quality of life	6.78/10
Status Index	n.a.
Management Index	n.a.
Majority religion	Catholicism
Traditional vs rational values [−2 to 2]	0.73
Survival vs self-expression values [−2 to 2]	0.36
Political structure	Regionalized
Corruption Perception Index	6.1/10
Population	0.41%
GDP per capita	84
Income level	17,600€/year
Unemployment rate	8.2%
Unemployment rate (youth)	15.7%
At risk poverty rate after social transfers	12.7%
GINI Index	23.8
Human Development Index	0.9

Policy factors	
Location regarding trafficking	Traffic country
Main drug trafficked	n.a.
Alcohol consumption—recorded	12.2
Alcohol consumption—unrecorded	15.19
Tobacco consumption—% of smokers	34.6%
Tobacco consumption—cigarettes per day	17.2
Cannabis prevalence all adults 15–64	3.1
Cannabis prevalence young adults 15–34	6.9
Cannabis prevalence youth 15–24	7.3
Heroin prevalence [lower/higher]	6.63/9.2
FCTC ratification year	2005
Party to the 1961 Single Convention	−
Party to the 1961 Single Convention as amended in 1972	1992

Annex 30: (continued) Slovenia—model 3

Ratification of 1971 Convention on Psychotropic Substances	1992
Party to the 1988 Convention	1992
National public spending on drug-related activities—% of GDP	0.03%
Strategy	
Responsible ministry for drug and addictions policies	Ministry of Health
The drug classification of the country determines the final penalties	No
Penalties for possessing drugs are higher than the EU recommendations	No
Penalties for trafficking drugs are higher than the EU recommendations	No
This country decriminalizes drug possession	No
Injection rooms—proxy for harm reduction	No
Alcohol policy scale	81/133
Alcohol price	84/234
Adopted written national policy on alcohol	Yes
Tobacco control scale	44/100
Specific national government objectives in tobacco control	Yes
Public health is included in the national strategy	No
Well-being is included in the national strategy	No
The country has EMCDDA best practices	No
Priority in the national strategy	Monitoring
Structure	
Ad hoc organization	Yes
Tackles legal and illicit substances together	No
Number of ministries involved	9/12
The country devolves policy-making to decentralized structures	Yes
The country devolves implementation to decentralized structures	Yes
Non-profit organization in the decision-making	No
Private organization in the implementation	No
Addiction is a priority in the national strategy	No
Year of the first law on illicit substances	2005

Data source: see Annex 5: Variables for factors construct and their definitions.

Annex 31: Spain—model 4

State factors	
Year of entry into the EU	1986
OECD Better Life Initiative	6/10
OECD material living conditions	4.93/10
OECD quality of life	7.08/10
Status Index	6.35/10
Management Index	6.03/10
Majority religion	Catholicism
Traditional vs rational values [–2 to 2]	0.09
Survival vs self-expression values [–2 to 2]	0.54
Political structure	Regionalized
Corruption Perception Index	6.2/10
Population	9.28%
GDP per capita	99
Income level	23,100€/year
Unemployment rate	21.7%
Unemployment rate (youth)	46.4%
At risk poverty rate after social transfers	20.7%
GINI Index	34
Human Development Index	0.9

Policy factors	
Location regarding trafficking	Entry point
Main drug trafficked	Cannabis and cocaine
Alcohol consumption—recorded	10.2
Alcohol consumption—unrecorded	11.62
Tobacco consumption—% of smokers	28.1%
Tobacco consumption—cigarettes per day	13.9
Cannabis prevalence all adults 15–64	10.6
Cannabis prevalence young adults 15–34	19.4
Cannabis prevalence youth 15–24	23.9
Heroin prevalence [lower/higher]	1.2/1.3
FCTC ratification year	2005
Party to the 1961 Single Convention	1961
Party to the 1961 Single Convention as amended in 1972	1977

Annex 31: (continued) Spain—model 4

Ratification of 1971 Convention on Psychotropic Substances	1973
Party to the 1988 Convention	1988
National public spending on drug-related activities—% of GDP	0.04%

Strategy

Responsible ministry for drug and addictions policies	Ministry of Health and Social Affairs
The drug classification of the country determines the final penalties	Yes
Penalties for possessing drugs are higher than the EU recommendations	Yes
Penalties for trafficking drugs are higher than the EU recommendations	Yes
This country decriminalizes drug possession	Yes
Injection rooms—proxy for harm reduction	Yes
Alcohol policy scale	54/133
Alcohol price	97/234
Adopted written national policy on alcohol	Yes
Tobacco control scale	46/100
Specific national government objectives in tobacco control	Yes
Public health is included in the national strategy	No
Well-being is included in the national strategy	No
The country has EMCDDA best practices	1, 2, & 3
Priority in the national strategy	Demand reduction

Structure

Ad hoc organization	Yes
Tackles legal and illicit substances together	Yes
Number of ministries involved	7/13
The country devolves policy-making to decentralized structures	Yes
The country devolves implementation to decentralized structures	Yes
Non-profit organization in the decision-making	No
Private organization in the implementation	No
Addiction is a priority in the national strategy	No
Year of the first law on illicit substances	1978

Data source: see Annex 5: Variables for factors construct and their definitions.

Annex 32: Sweden—model 2

State factors

Year of entry into the EU	1995
OECD Better Life Initiative	7.3/10
OECD material living conditions	6.23/10
OECD quality of life	8.38/10
Status Index	8.65/10
Management Index	8.29/10
Majority religion	Protestantism
Traditional vs rational values [–2 to 2]	1.86
Survival vs self-expression values [–2 to 2]	2.35
Political structure	Unitary
Corruption Perception Index	9.3/10
Population	1.85%
GDP per capita	126
Income level	41,100€/year
Unemployment rate	7.5%
Unemployment rate (youth)	22.9%
At risk poverty rate after social transfers	12.9%
GINI Index	24.4
Human Development Index	0.9

Policy factors

Location regarding trafficking	Transit and final destination
Main drug trafficked	n.a.
Alcohol consumption—recorded	6.7
Alcohol consumption—unrecorded	10.3
Tobacco consumption—% of smokers	16%
Tobacco consumption—cigarettes per day	10.1
Cannabis prevalence all adults 15–64	2.8
Cannabis prevalence young adults 15–34	6.2
Cannabis prevalence youth 15–24	7.3
Heroin prevalence [lower/higher]	n.a.
FCTC ratification year	2005
Party to the 1961 Single Convention	1961

Annex 32: (continued) Sweden—model 2

Party to the 1961 Single Convention as amended in 1972	1972
Ratification of 1971 Convention on Psychotropic Substances	1972
Party to the 1988 Convention	1991
National public spending on drug-related activities—% of GDP	0.17–0.39%

Strategy

Responsible ministry for drug and addictions policies	Ministry of Health
The drug classification of the country determines the final penalties	No
Penalties for possessing drugs are higher than the EU recommendations	No
Penalties for trafficking drugs are higher than the EU recommendations	Yes
This country decriminalizes drug possession	No
Injection rooms—proxy for harm reduction	No
Alcohol policy scale	124/133
Alcohol price	138/234
Adopted written national policy on alcohol	Yes
Tobacco control scale	51/100
Specific national government objectives in tobacco control	Yes
Public health is included in the national strategy	No
Well-being is included in the national strategy	No
The country has EMCDDA best practices	1 & 2
Priority in the national strategy	Prevention

Structure

Ad hoc organization	Yes
Tackles legal and illicit substances together	Yes
Number of ministries involved	4/12
The country devolves policy-making to decentralized structures	Yes
The country devolves implementation to decentralized structures	Yes
Non-profit organization in the decision-making	Yes
Private organization in the implementation	Yes
Addiction is a priority in the national strategy	No
Year of the first law on illicit substances	1968

Data source: see Annex 5: Variables for factors construct and their definitions.

Annex 33: UK—model 2

State factors	
Year of entry into the EU	1973
OECD Better Life Initiative	7.2/10
OECD material living conditions	6.7/10
OECD quality of life	7.7/10
Status Index	7.22/10
Management Index	6.82/10
Majority religion	Protestantism and Catholicism
Traditional vs rational values [–2 to 2]	0.06
Survival vs self-expression values [–2 to 2]	1.68
Political structure	Unitary
Corruption Perception Index	8.6/10
Population	12.28%
GDP per capita	108
Income level	27,900€/year
Unemployment rate	8%
Unemployment rate (youth)	21.1%
At risk poverty rate after social transfers	17.1%
GINI Index	33
Human Development Index	0.9
Policy factors	
Location regarding trafficking	Final destination
Main drug trafficked	Cannabis and heroin
Alcohol consumption—recorded	11.7
Alcohol consumption—unrecorded	13.37
Tobacco consumption—% of smokers	26.7%
Tobacco consumption—cigarettes per day	14.6
Cannabis prevalence all adults 15–64	8.4
Cannabis prevalence young adults 15–34	15.9
Cannabis prevalence youth 15–24	21.2
Heroin prevalence [lower/higher]	2.86/5.76
FCTC ratification year	2004
Party to the 1961 Single Convention	1961

Annex 33: (continued) UK—model 2

Party to the 1961 Single Convention as amended in 1972	1978
atification of 1971 Convention on Psychotropic Substances	1971
Party to the 1988 Convention	1988
National public spending on drug-related activities—% of GDP	0.08%

Strategy

Responsible ministry for drug and addictions policies	Home Office (Ministry of Interior)
The drug classification of the country determines the final penalties	Yes
Penalties for possessing drugs are higher than the EU recommendations	Yes
Penalties for trafficking drugs are higher than the EU recommendations	Yes
This country decriminalizes drug possession	No
Injection rooms—proxy for harm reduction	No
Alcohol policy scale	79/133
Alcohol price	117/234
Adopted written national policy on alcohol	Yes
Tobacco control scale	77/100
Specific national government objectives in tobacco control	Yes
Public health is included in the national strategy	No
Well-being is included in the national strategy	No
The country has EMCDDA best practices	1, 2, & 3
Priority in the national strategy	Demand reduction

Structure

Ad hoc organization	Yes
Tackles legal and illicit substances together	No
Number of ministries involved	15/22
The country devolves policy-making to decentralized structures	Yes
The country devolves implementation to decentralized structures	Yes
Non-profit organization in the decision-making	Yes
Private organization in the implementation	Yes
Addiction is a priority in the national strategy	No
Year of the first law on illicit substances	1971

Data source: see Annex 5: Variables for factors construct and their definitions.

Bibliography

Abellán, L. (2012) Bruselas obligará a cubrir la cajetilla de tabaco con imágenes disuasorias [online journal] <http://sociedad.elpais.com/sociedad/2012/12/19/actualidad/1355924436_650998.html> (accessed 18 July 2013).

Advisory Council on the Misuse of Drugs (1988) AIDS and drug misuse. London: HMSO.

Advisory Council on the Misuse of Drugs (2012) [website] <https://www.gov.uk/government/organizations/advisory-council-on-the-misuse-of-drugs> (accessed 18 July 2013).

Agranoff, R. (2012) Collaborating to Manage. Washington, D.C: Georgetown University Press.

Ahlquist, J. S. and Breunig, C. (2011) Model-based clustering and typologies in the social sciences. Political Analysis 20: 92–112.

Ahlström, S. K. and Österberg, E. L. (2005) International perspectives on adolescent and young drinking. Alcohol Research and Health 28: 258–268.

Albareda L., Lozano J. M., and Ysa T. (2007) Public policies on corporate social responsibility: The Role of Governments in Europe. Journal of Business Ethics 74: 391–407.

Alcohol Abuse Among Adolescents in Europe (2012) [website] <http://www.aaaprevent.eu/> (accessed 18 July 2013).

Alcohol Policy UK (2012) Government's Alcohol Strategy: 2012 national strategy confirms minimum pricing for England and Wales [website] <http://www.alcoholpolicy.net/2012/03/national-alcohol-strategy-2012-government-alcohol-strategy-choice-challenge-and-responsibility-confi.html> (accessed 20 July 2013).

Alcohol Policy UK (2013) Government confirms no minimum pricing or multi-buy ban as health groups left reeling [website] <http://www.alcoholpolicy.net/2013/07/government-confirms-no-minimum-pricing-or-ban-on-multi-buy-deals-as-health-groups-left-reeling.html?utm_source=feedburner&utm_medium=feed&utm_campaign=Feed%3A+AlcoholPolicyUk+%28Alcohol+Policy+UK%29> (accessed 20 July 2013).

ALICE RAP (2012) Alcohol—the neglected addiction. ALICE RAP policy papers series. Policy Brief 1.

American Society of Addiction Medicine (2012) [website] <http://www.asam.org> (accessed 18 July 2013).

Amphora (2012) The Amphora manifesto on alcohol. Amphora Project (2009–2012). European Commission 7th Framework Program.

Anderson, P., Moller, L., and Galea, G. (2012) Alcohol in the European Union: Consumption, harm and policy approaches. Copenhagen: World Health Organization Regional Office for Europe.

Arif, A. (1981) Los problemas de la droga en el mundo y las estrategias de la OMS, in G. Edwards and A. Arif (eds), Los problemas de la droga en el contexto sociocultural. Una base para la formulación de políticas y la planificación de programas. Ginebra: OMS, pp. 22–35.

Armyr, G., Elmér, Å., and Herz, U. (1982) Alcohol in the world of the 80s: Habits, attitudes, preventive policies and voluntary efforts. Stockholm: Sober Förlag AB.

Arts, W. and Gelissen, J. (2002) Three worlds of welfare capitalism of more? Journal of European Social Policy **12**: 137–158.

Austria—EMCDDA Country Overview (2011) [website] <http://www.emcdda.europa.eu/publications/country-overviews/at> (accessed 18 July 2013).

Babor, R., Caetano, S., Casswell, G., et al. (2010). Alcohol: No ordinary commodity. Research and public policy. Oxford: Oxford University Press.

Baltic News Network (2012) Illicit alcohol market proportion in Latvia is nearly 40%. Baltic News Network [online journal] <http://bnn-news.com/illicit-alcohol-market-proportion-latvia-40-72712> (accessed 18 July 2013).

BBC News (2007) Baltic neighbours face alcohol crisis. BBC News [online journal] <http://news.bbc.co.uk/2/hi/europe/6957153.stm> (accessed 18 July 2013).

Beblavý, M. (2008) New welfare state models based on the new member states' experience? Stream 4 Comparative methodology: worlds and varieties of welfare capitalism. Social Governance Institute.

Bekke, A. J. G. M. and Meer, F. M. (2000) Civil service systems in Western Europe. Northampton, MA: Edward Elgar Publishing.

Belgium Drug Policy Note (2011) Note politique du Gouvernement fédéral relative à la problématique de la drogue.

Belgium—EMCDDA Country Overview (2011) [website] <http://www.emcdda.europa.eu/publications/country-overviews/be> (accessed 18 July 2013).

Bergeron, H. and Griffiths, P. (2006) Drifting towards a more common approach to a more common problem: epidemiology and the evolution of European drug policy, in R. Hughes, R. Lart, and P. Higate (eds), Drugs: policy and politics. London: Open University Press, pp. 113–124.

Berridge, V. and Mars, S. (2004) History of addictions. Journal of Epidemiology & Community Health **58**: 747–750.

Bertelsmann Stiftung (2011) [website] <http://www.sgi-network.org/> (accessed 18 July 2013).

Bewley-Taylor, D. R. (2012) International drug control: consensus fractured. Cambridge: Cambridge University Press.

Bohle, D. and Greskovits, B. (2006) Capitalism without compromise: strong business and weak labor in Eastern Europe's new transational industries. Studies in Comparative International Development **41**: 3–25.

Bongers, I. M. B., van de Goor, I. A. M., and Garretsen, H. F. L. (1998) Social climate on alcohol in Rotterdam, the Netherlands: public opinion on drinking behavior and alcohol control measures. Alcohol & Alcoholism **32**: 141–150.

Bouso, J. C. (2003) Qué son las drogas de síntesis. Madrid: RBA Integra.

Bovaird, T. (2004) Public private partnerships: from contested concepts to prevalent practice. International Review of Administrative Science **70**: 199–215.

Braun, D. and Gilardi, F. (2006) Taking 'Galton's problem' seriously: Towards a theory of policy diffusion. Journal of Theoretical Politics **18**: 298–322.

Brown, M. M., Dewar, M. F., and Wallace, P. (1982). International survey: Alcoholic beverage taxation and control policies. Ottawa: Brewers Association of Canada.

Brun-Gulbrandsen, S. (1988) Drinking habits in Norway, in O. J. Skog, and R. Waahlberg (eds), Alcohol and drugs: The Norwegian experience. Oslo: National Directorate for the Prevention of Alcohol and Drug Problems, pp. 13–28.

Bulgaria—EMCDDA Country Overview (2011) [website] <http://www.emcdda.europa.eu/publications/country-overviews/bg> (accessed 18 July 2013).

Bulgaria National Drug Strategy (2009) National Strategy for combating drugs. Republic of Bulgaria.

Bunyan, T. (1993). Statewatching the new Europe: A handbook on the European state. London: Statewatch Publication/UNISON.

Burning, E. C. (1991) Effects of Amsterdam needle and syringe exchange. International Journal of Mental Health and Addiction **26**: 1303–1311.

CAMH Knowledge Exchange (2010) Primary care addiction toolkit [website], <http://knowledgex.camh.net/primary_care/toolkits/addiction_toolkit/fundamentals/Pages/faq_dependence_tolerance.aspx#dependence> (accessed 18 July 2013).

Camilleri, I. (2010) [website] <http://www.timesofmalta.com/articles/view/20100423/local/vast-majority-want-ban-on-alcohol-for-under-18-year-olds.304040> (accessed 18 July 2013).

Carnwath, T. and Smith, I. (2002). Heroin century. London: Routledge.

Caudevilla, F. (2007). Éxtasis (MDMA). Madrid: Amargord.

Central Intelligence Agency (2012) [website] <https://www.cia.gov> (accessed 18 July 2013).

Cerami, A. (2006) Social policy in Central and Eastern Europe: The emergence of a new European welfare regime. Berlin: LIT Verlag.

Chatwin, C. (2007) Multi-level governance: The way forward for European illicit drug policy? International Journal of Drug Policy **18**: 494–502.

Colom, J. (2001) Análisis de las intervenciones en drogodependencias en el Estado Español desde sus orígenes hasta la reducción de daños. Barcelona: Grup IGIA.

Comas, D. (1985) El uso de las drogas en la juventud. Madrid: Instituto de la Juventud.

Comas, D. (1988) El tratamiento de la drogodependencia y las comunidades terapéuticas. Madrid: PNSD.

Comas, D. (1989) La construcción social de la imagen del drogodependiente: consecuencias para la prevención y atención, in Jornada de Psicología de la intervención social. Madrid: Inserso, pp. 233–261.

Comelles, J. M. and Martínez, A. (1993) Enfermedad, cultura y sociedad. Madrid: Eudema.

Committee of Inquiry into the Drugs Problem in the Member States of the Community (1986) chaired by Sir Jack Stewart-Clark MEP (OJ C283, 10 November).

Cooney, P. (1992) Report drawn up by the Committee of Enquiry into the spread of organised crime linked to drugs trafficking in the Member States of the European Community. Issues 358–391 of European Parliament session documents. European Parliament.

Council of the European Communities (1989) Council Directive 89/552/EEC on the Coordination of certain provisions laid down by law, regulation or administrative action in Member States concerning the pursuit of television broadcasting activities. 89/552/EEC

Council of the European Communities (1992a) Council Directive 92/84/EEC of 19 October 1992 on the approximation of the rates of excise duty on alcohol and alcoholic beverages.

Council of the European Communities (1992b) Council Regulation (EEC) No 2075/92 of 30 June 1992 on the common organization of the market in raw tobacco.

Council of the European Communities (1992c) Council Directive 92/85/EEC of 19 October 1992 on the introduction of measures to encourage improvements in the safety and health at work of pregnant workers and workers who have recently given birth or are breastfeeding (tenth individual Directive within the meaning of Article 16 (1) of Directive 89/391/EEC).

Council of the European Communities (1993) Council Regulation (EEC) No 302/93 of 8 February 1993 on the establishment of a European Monitoring Centre for Drugs and Drug Addiction.

Council of the EU (1996) Council Resolution of 26 November 1996 on the reduction of smoking in the European Community (96(C 374/04).

Council of the EU (1999) European Union Drugs Strategy (2000–2004). 12555/3/99 REV3.

Council of the EU (2001) Directive 2001/37/EC of the European Parliament and the Council of 5 June 2001 on the approximation of the laws, regulations and administrative provisions of the Member States concerning the manufacture, presentation and sale of tobacco products. Luxembourg, 5 June 2001.

Council of the EU (2002) Action plan on Drugs between the EU and Central Asian republics (Kazakhstan, Kyrgyzstan, Tajikistan, Uzbekistan). 12353/02.

Council of the EU (2003a) Council Decision of 19 December 2002 establishing criteria and procedures for the acceptance of waste at landfills pursuant to Article 16 of and Annex II to Directive 1999/31/EC. Brussels, 19 December 2002.

Council of the EU (2003b). Draft Action Plan on Drugs between the EU and Countries of Western Balkans and Candidate Countries (Bulgaria, Romania and Turkey). 5062/2/03 REV2 COR1.

Council of the EU (2004a). EU Drugs Strategy (2005–2012). 15074/04 CORDROGUE 77.

Council of the EU (2004b) Council Framework Decision 2004/757/JHA of 25 October 2004 laying down minimum provisions on the constituent elements of criminal acts and penalties in the field of illicit drug trafficking.

Council of the EU (2004c) Draft Council Resolution on Cannabis. 11267/04. CORDROGUE 59. Brussels, 7 July 2004

Council of the EU (2005) EU Drugs Action Plan (2005–2008). 2005/C 168/01.

Council of the EU (2006a) Action oriented paper on implementing with Russia the common space of freedom, security and justice. 15534/1/06.

Council of the EU (2006b) Action oriented aper increasing EU support for combating drug production in and trafficking from Afghanistan, including transit routes. 9370/1/06.

Council of the EU (2007) Directive 2007/65/EC of the European Parliament and the Council of 11 December 2007 amending Council Directive 89/552/EEC on the coordination of certain provisions laid down by law, regulation or administrative action in Member States concerning the pursuit of television broadcasting activities. Strasbourg, 11 December 2007.

Council of the EU (2008) EU Drugs Action Plan for 2009-2012. 2008/C 326/09.

Council of the EU (2009a) Draft Action Plan on drugs between the EU and the Western Balkan countries (2009–2013). 12185/09.

Council of the EU (2009b) 2009–2013 Action plan on Drugs between the EU and Central Asian states. 9961/09.

Council of the EU (2010a) Council Directive 2010/12/EU of 16 February 2010 amending Directives 92/79/EEC, 92/80/EEC and 95/59/EC on the structure and rates of excise duty applied on manufactured tobacco and Directive 2008/118/EC. Brussels, 16 February 2010.

Council of the EU (2010b) European pact to combat international drug trafficking—disrupting cocaine and heroin routes. 3018th JUSTICE and HOME AFFAIRS Council meeting.

Council of the EU (2011). EU-Western Balkans dialogue on drugs. 10860/11.

Council of the EU (2012) Council conclusions on the new EU drugs strategy. 3172nd Justice and Home Affairs Council meeting.

Courtwright, D. T. (2001). Las drogas y la formación del mundo moderno. Barcelona: Paidós.

Cyprus—EMCDDA Country Overview (2011) [website] <http://www.emcdda.europa.eu/publications/country-overviews/cy> (accessed 18 July 2013).

Cyprus National Strategy on Drugs 2009–2012 (2009) Cyprus Antidrugs Council.

Czech National Drug Policy Strategy for the Period 2010–2018 (2010) Government Resolution N. 340.

Czech Republic—EMCDDA Country Overview (2011) [website] <http://www.emcdda.europa.eu/publications/country-overviews/cz> (accessed 18 July 2013).

Czech Republic—EMCDDA Drug Treatment Profile (2011) [website] <http://www.emcdda.europa.eu/html.cfm/index35879EN.html> (accessed 18 July 2013).

Dapkus, L. and Peach, G. (2008) Exit poll: conservatives ahead in Lithuania vote. Fox News [online journal] <http://www.foxnews.com/printer_friendly_wires/2008Oct12/0,4675,EULithuaniaElections,00.html> (accessed 18 July 2013).

Davies, P. and Walsh, D. (1983) Alcohol problems and alcohol control in Europe. New York: Gardner Press.

De Benito, E. (2010) Más drogadictos legales. El País [online journal] <http://elpais.com/diario/2010/12/08/sociedad/1291762801_850215.html> (accessed 18 July 2013).

De Frel, J. (2009) Welfare state classification: The development of Central Eastern European welfare states. PhD thesis (Erasmus University, Rotterdam).

Deacon, B. (1993) Developments in East European social policy, in C. Jones (ed.), New perspectives on the welfare state in Europe. London: Routledge, pp. 163–183.

Del Olmo, R. (1987) La cara oculta de la droga. Poder y control 2: 23–48.

Denmark Action Plan (2010) Kampen mod narko II Handlingsplan mod narkotikamisbrug. Danish Government.

Denmark—EMCDDA Country Overview (2011) [website] <http://www.emcdda.europa.eu/publications/country-overviews/dk> (accessed 18 July 2013).

Deprez, N., Antoine, J., Asueta-Lorente, et al. (2011) Belgian national report on drugs. EMCDDA.

Des Larlais, D. C. (1995) Harm reduction: A framework for incorporating science into drug policy. American Journal of Public Health 85: 10–12.

Dias, L. (2007) As drogas em Portugal: o fenómeno e os factos jurídico-políticos de 1970 a 2004. Coimbra: Pé de Página Editores.

Díaz, A. (1998) Hoja, pasta, polvo, roca. El consumo de los derivados de la coca. Bellatera: Servei de Publicacions de la UAB.

Díaz, A., Barruti, M., and Doncel, C. (1992) Les línies de l'èxit? Naturalesa i extensió del consum de cocaïna a Barcelona. Barcelona: Ajuntament de Barcelona.

Díaz, A., Pallarés, J., Barruti M., et al. (2004) Observatori de nous consums de drogues en l'àmbit juvenil. Barcelona: Institut Genus.

Drug Commissioner of the Federal Government [of Germany] (2012) National Strategy on Drug and Addiction Policy [website] <http://drogenbeauftragte.de/fileadmin/dateien-dba/Presse/Downloads/Nationale_Strategie_Druckfassung_EN.pdf> (accessed 7 August 2013).

Elder, M. (2008) Smugglers built vodka pipeline. Telegraph [online journal] <http://www.telegraph.co.uk/news/worldnews/europe/russia/2975934/Smugglers-built-vodka-pipeline.html> (accessed 18 July 2013).

Elvins, M. (2003) Anti-drugs policies of the European Union: Transnational decision-making and the politics of expertise. Hampshire: Palgrave Macmillan.

EMCDDA (2003) The state of the drugs problem in the acceding and candidate countries to the European Union. EMCDDA Annual Report 2003.

EMCDDA (2005) Illicit drug use in the EU: legislative approaches. EMCDDA Thematic Papers.

EMCDDA (2008a) Monitoring the supply of heroin in Europe. EMCDDA Technical Data Sheets.

EMCDDA (2008b) A cannabis reader: global issues and local experiences Perspectives on cannabis controversies, treatment and regulation in Europe. EMCDDA Monographs.

EMCDDA (2010) Statistical bulletin [website] <http://www.emcdda.europa.eu/stats10> (accessed 18 July 2013).

EMCDDA (2011a) Annual report 2011: The state of the drugs problem in Europe. EMCDDA Annual Reports.

EMCDDA (2011b) Statistical bulletin—2011 [website] <http://www.emcdda.europa.eu/stats11> (accessed 18 July 2013).

EMCDDA (2011c) Best Practice Portal. [website] <http://www.emcdda.europa.eu/best-practice> (accessed 18 July 2013).

EMCDDA (2013a) Hungary—National drug-related information data [website], <http://www.emcdda.europa.eu/countries/public-expenditure/hungary> (accessed 18 July 2013).

EMCDDA (2013b) European drug report–trends and analysis. Lisbon: EMCDDA.

EMCDDA (2013c) Statistical bulletin [website] <http://www.emcdda.europa.eu/stats13> (accessed 18 July 2013).

EMCDDA (2013d) Key EU activities on drugs—chronology [website] <http://www.emcdda.europa.eu/html.cfm/index2982EN.html> (accessed 18 July 2013).

EMCDDA and Europol (2011) Annual report on the implementation of Council Decision 2005/387/JHA. EMCDDA Implementation Reports.

EMCDDA and Europol (2012) EMCDDA–Europol 2011 Annual Report on the implementation of Council Decision 2005/387/JHA In accordance with Article 10 of Council Decision 2005/387/JHA on the information exchange, risk assessment and control of new psychoactive substances.

EMCDDA and SNIPH (2011) 2012 National Report (2011 data) to the EMCDDA by the Reitox National Focal Point: Sweden New Development, Trends and in-depth information on selected issues. REITOX.

Emerson, K., Nabatchi, T., and Balogh, S. (2012) An integrative framework for collaborative governance. Journal of Public Administration Research Theory **22**: 1–31.

Eriksen, M., Mackay, J., and Ross, H. (2012) The tobacco atlas: Fourth edition completely revised and updated. Atlanta: American Cancer Society.

Escohotado. A. (1989) Historia general de las drogas. Alianza: Madrid.

Esping-Andersen, G. (1990) The three worlds of welfare capitalism. Oxford: Polity Press.

Esping-Andersen, G. (1993) The comparative macro-sociology of welfare states, in L. Moreno (ed.), Social exchange and welfare development. Madrid: Consejo Superior de Investigaciones Científicas, pp. 123–136.

Esping-Andersen, G. (1994) Welfare states and the economy, in N. J. Smelser and R. Swedberg (eds), The handbook of economic sociology. Princeton/New York: Princeton University Press/Russel Sage Foundation, pp. 711–732.

Esping-Andersen, G. (1996a) Welfare states without work: The impasse of labour shedding and familialism in continental European social policy, in G. Esping-Andersen (ed.), Welfare states in transition. London: Sage, pp. 66–87.

Esping-Andersen, G. (1996b) Welfare states in transition: National adaptations in global economies. London: Sage.

Esping-Andersen, G. (1997) Hybrid or Unique? The Japanese Welfare State between Europe and America', Journal of European Social Policy 7:179–189.

Esping-Andersen, G. (1999) Social foundations of post-industrial economies. Oxford: Oxford University Press.

Esping-Andersen, G. and Korpi, W. (1984) Social policy as class politics in post-war capitalism, in J. Goldthorpe (ed.), Order and conflict in contemporary capitalism. Oxford: Oxford University Press, pp. 179–208.

Esteve, M., Boyne, G., Sierra, V., et al. (2012a) Organizational collaboration in the public sector: Do chief executives make a difference? Journal of Public Administration Research and Theory 23(4): 927–952.

Esteve, M., Ysa, T., and Longo, F. (2012b) the creation of innovation through public-private collaboration. Revista Española de Cardiología 65(9): 835–842.

Estonia—EMCDDA Country Overview (2011) [website] <http://www.emcdda.europa.eu/publications/country-overviews/ee> (accessed 18 July 2013).

Estonian Public Broadcasting (2011) [website] Nation Suffering From Highest Rate of Drug-Related Deaths in EU. <http://news.err.ee/v/society/780d730b-e6f2-4b79-a38c-8088367a7811> (accessed 17 February 2014).

EurActiv (2006) Industry opposes EU alcohol strategy. EurActiv [online journal] <http://www.euractiv.com/health/industry-opposes-eu-alcohol-strategy/article-156818> (accessed 18 July 2013).

Europa Summaries of EU Legislation (2012) [website] <http://europa.eu/legislation_summaries/public_health/health_determinants_lifestyle/c11577_en.htm> (accessed 18 July 2013).

European Centre for Disease Prevention and Control—WHO Regional Office for Europe (2010) HIV/AIDS surveillance in Europe 2009. Stockholm: European Centre for Disease Prevention and Control.

European Coalition for Just and Effective Drug Policies (2012) No more time to waste, prohibition has failed. ENCOD Bulletin N. 88 on Drug Policies in Europe.

EC (1999) Report from the Commission to the Council, the European Parliament and Social Committee and the Committee of the Regions: Progress achieved in relation to public health protection from the harmful effects of tobacco consumption. COM (99) 407 final. Brussels, 08.09.1999.

EC (2006a) An EU strategy to support Member States in reducing alcohol related harm. Communication from the Commission to the Council, the European Parliament, the European Economic and Social Committee and the Committee of the Regions. COM(2006) yyy final.

EC (2006b) Green Paper on the role of Civil Society in Drugs Policy in the European Union. COM(2006) **316** final.

EC (2007a) Report on the Green Paper Consultation: Towards a Europe free from tobacco smoke: policy option at EU level. European Commission & DG Health and Consumer Protection.

EC (2007b) Charter Establishing the European Alcohol and Health Forum.

EC (2008) Report Final Evaluation of the EU Drugs Action Plan (2005-2008) SEC(2008) 2456.

EC (2009) Eurobarometer 72.3: Tobacco. Special Eurobarometer 332.

EC (2011) Action plan to fight against smuggling of cigarettes and alcohol along the EU Eastern border. SEC(2011) 791 final Commission Anti-fraud Strategy.

EC (2012) Proposal for a Directive of the European Parliament and of the Council on the approximation of the laws, regulations and administrative provisions of the Member States concerning the manufacture, presentation and sale of tobacco and related products. COM(2012) 788 final. Brussels, 19.12.2012.

EC–DG Health (2011) [website] <http://ec.europa.eu/health/alcohol/forum/> (accessed 18 July 2013).

EC—DG Agriculture and Rural Development (2012) [website] <http://ec.europa.eu/agriculture/markets/tobacco/index_en.htm> (accessed 18 July 2013).

EC—DG Health (2012) [website] <http://ec.europa.cu/health/tobacco/introduction/index_en.htm> (accessed 18 July 2013).

EC—DG Justice (2011) [website] <http://ec.europa.eu/justice/anti-drugs/civil-society/index_en.htm> (accessed 18 July 2013).

EC—DG Justice (2012) [website] <http://ec.europa.eu/justice/anti-drugs/situation-europe/index_en.htm> (accessed 18 July 2013).

EU (2010) Treaty on the Functioning of the European Union. Official Journal of the European Union, Article 288.

European Voice (1997) MEPs demand 'alcopop' controls. Eurpean Voice. <http://www.europeanvoice.com/article/imported/meps-demand-alcopop-controls/33837.aspx> (accessed 18 July 2013).

Europol (2011) EU organized crime threat assessment (OCTA 2011) Analysis & Knowledge. The Hague: European Police Office.

Europol (2012) [website] <https://www.europol.europa.eu/content/page/europol%E2%80%99s-priorities-145> (accessed 18 July 2013).

Eurostat (2011a) [website] <http://epp.eurostat.ec.europa.eu> (accessed 18 July 2013).

Eurostat (2011b) Gini coefficient [website] <http://appsso.eurostat.ec.europa.eu/nui/show.do?dataset=ilc_di12&lang=en> (accessed 18 July 2013).

Eurostat (2011c) Unemployment Statistics [website] <http://epp.eurostat.ec.europa.eu/statistics_explained/index.php/Unemployment_statistics> (accessed 18 July 2013).

Faid, M. and Gleicher, D. (2011) Dancing the tango: the experience and roles of the European Union in relation to the Framework Convention on Tobacco Control. Geneva: Global Health Europe and the Graduate Institute, Geneva Global Health Program.

Ferrera, M. (1996) The 'southern' model of welfare in social Europe. Journal of European Social Policy **6**: 17–37.

Finnish Ministry of Social Affairs and Health (1994) The Alcohol Act: 1143/1994, Government of Finland, 8 December 1994.

Finland—EMCDDA Country Overview (2011) [website] <http://www.emcdda.europa.eu/publications/country-overviews/fi> (accessed 18 July 2013).

Foucault. M. (1963) El nacimiento de la clínica. México: Siglo XXI.

France—EMCDDA and OFDT National Report (2012) 2011 National Report (2010 data) to the EMCDDA by the Reitox National Focal Point France New Development, Trends and in-depth information on selected issues. REITOX.

France—EMCDDA and OFDT National Report (2011) 2010 National Report (2009 data) to the EMCDDA by the Reitox National Focal Point France New Development, Trends and in-depth information on selected issues. REITOX.

France—EMCDDA Country Overview (2011) [website] <http://www.emcdda.europa.eu/publications/country-overviews/fr> (accessed 18 July 2013).

French Inter-departmental Mission for the Fight against Drugs and Drug Addiction—MILDT (2008) French Governmental Plan to fight against drugs and drug addiction. Premier ministre, République Française.

Gamella, J. F. (1992) La historia de Julián. Madrid: Popular.

García Prado, G. (2002) Los años de la aguja: Del compromiso político a la heroína. Zaragoza: Mira Editores.

Garretsen, H. F. L. and Knibbe, R. A. (1985) Alcohol consumption and alcohol control policy: the case of the Netherlands. Health Policy **5**: 151–158.

Georgiev, V. (2010) Towards a common European border security policy. European Security **19**: 255–274.

German Action Plan on Drugs and Addiction (2003) German Ministry of Health and Social Security.

Germany—EMCDDA Country Overview (2011) <http://www.emcdda.europa.eu/publications/country-overviews/de>.

Gil Muñoz, C. (1970) Juventud Marginada. Un estudio sobre los hippies a su paso por Formentera. Barcelona: Dopesa.

Global Post (2010) Prague: The new Amsterdam? Global Post: America's world news site [online journal] <http://www.globalpost.com/dispatch/czech-republic/101127/marijuana-laws> (accessed 18 July 2013).

Götz, W. (2012) Opening address in the Global forum on combating illicit drug trafficking and related threats. World Customs Organization.

Government of Finland (2008) Finnish Resolution on Drug Policy Co-operation for the years 2008–2011.

Government of Malta (2012) [website] <https://gov.mt> (accessed 18 July 2013).

Government of Romania (2005) Romanian National Anti-drug Strategy 2005–2012.

Government of the Slovak Republic (2009) Slovakian national anti-drug strategy for the period 2009–2012.

Greece—EMCDDA Country Overview (2011) [website] <http://www.emcdda.europa.eu/publications/country-overviews/el> (accessed 18 July 2013).

Greece—EMCDDA Legal Profile (2011) [website] <http://www.emcdda.europa.eu/html.cfm/index5174EN.html?pluginMethod=eldd.countryprofiles&country=GR> (accessed 18 July 2013).

Greece—EMCDDA, UMHRI and REITOX National Report (2010) 2010 National Report (2009 data) to the EMCDDA by the Reitox National Focal Point GREECE New Development, Trends and in-depth information on selected issues. REITOX.

Greenwald, G. (2009) Drug decriminalization in Portugal: Lessons for creating fair and successful drug policies. Cato Institute.

Greve, C. and Hodge, G. (2013) Rethingking Public-Private Partnerships. Strategies for Turbulent Times. Abingdon: Routledge.

Grup Igia (2000) Contextos sujetos y drogas: un manual sobre drogodependencias. Barcelona/Madrid: Ajuntament de Barcelona/FAD.

Hall, J., Giovannini, E., Morrone, A., et al. (2010) A framework to measure the progress of societies. OECD Statistics Working Papers, 2010/05. Paris: OECD Publishing.

Hall, P. A. and Soskice, D. (2001) Varieties of capitalism: The institutional foundations of comparative advantage. Oxford: Oxford University Press.

Harkin, A. M. (1995) Profiles of Alcohol in the Member States of the European Region of the World Health Organization. Copenhagen: WHO Regional Office for Europe.

Helsingin Sanomat (2010) [website] <http://www.hs.fi/> (accessed 18 July 2013).

Hidalgo, E. (2007) Heroína. Madrid: Amargord.

Hidalgo, E., Calzada, N. and Rovira, J. (2006) Programas de reducción de riesgos. Revista de Estudios Sobre Juventud 24: 90–109.

H.M. Government (2012) The government's alcohol strategy. London: Stationery Office.

Holder, H. D., Kühlhorn, E., Nordlund, S., et al. (1998) European integration and nordic alcohol policies. changes in alcohol control policies and consequences in Finland, Norway and Sweden, 1980-1997. Aldershot: Ashgate.

Holmberg, R. (2001) A review of the Swedish treatment system: IKB 1999. Nordisk alkohol & narkotikatidskrift 18: 190–197.

Hughes, C. and Stevens, A. (2010) What can we learn from the Portuguese decriminalization of illicit drugs. British Journal of Criminology s: 999–1022.

Hungarian National Assembly (2009) National Strategy to address the drug problem 2010-2018. Government of Hungary.

Hungary—EMCDDA Country Overview (2011) [website] <http://www.emcdda.europa.eu/publications/country-overviews/hu> (accessed 18 July 2013).

Hungary-EMCDDA National Drug Strategy (2012) [website]<http://www.emcdda.europa.eu/countries/national-drug-strategies/hungary> (accessed, 14 February 2014)

Hurst, W., Gregory, E., and Gussman, T. (1997) International survey: Alcoholic beverage taxation and control policies. 9th edn. Ottawa: Brewers Association of Canada.

Huxham, C. and Vangen, S. (2005) Managing to Collaborate. The theory and practice of collaborative advantage. Abingdon: Routledge.

Inglehart, R. and Welzel, C. (2005) Modernization, cultural change and democracy. New York: Cambridg University Press.

Inglehart, R. and Welzel, C. (2010) Changing mass priorities: the link between modernization and democracy. Perspectives on Politics 8: 551–567.

Institute of Alcohol Studies (2013) Government U-turn on minimum unit pricing of alcohol in England. *Globe* **3**: 8–9.

Institute on Drugs and Drug Addiction (2005) Portugal strategic plan against drugs and drug addiction 2005–2012. Ministry of Health of Portugal.

Institute on Drugs and Drug Addiction (2009) Portugal action plan 2009–2012. Ministry of Health of Portugal.

International Drug Policy Consortium (2008) The International Narcotic Control Board: Current tensions and options for reform. IDPC Briefing Paper 7.

International Drug Policy Consortium (2012) Informe IDPC-CGPD: Modernización del sistema mundial de fiscalización de estupefacientes—¿Puede Europa actuar como guía? Brussels: IDPC.

INCB (2012) [website] <http://www.incb.org> (accessed 18 July 2013).

Ireland—EMCDDA Country Overview (2011) [website] <http://www.emcdda.europa.eu/publications/country-overviews/ie> (accessed 18 July 2013).

Italian Action Plan on Drugs 2010–2013 (2010) Presidency of the Council of Ministers, Department of Antidrugs Policies.

Italy—EMCDDA Country Overview (2011) [website] <http://www.emcdda.europa.eu/publications/country-overviews/it> (accessed 18 July 2013).

Järvinen, M. and Room, R. (2007) Youth drinking cultures: European experiences, in M. Järvinen, and R. Room (eds), Youth drinking cultures: European experiences. Hampshire: Ashgate, pp. 1–17.

Joossens, L. and Raw, M. (2007) Progress in tobacco control in 30 European countries, 2005 to 2007. Berne: Swiss Cancer League.

Joossens, L. and Raw, M. (2010) The tobacco control scale 2010 in Europe. Brussels: Association of the European Cancer Leagues.

Joossens, L. and Raw, M. (2012) From cigarette smuggling to illicit tobacco trade. Tobacco Control **21**: 230–234.

Joossens L, M. D., and Ross, R. M. (2009) How eliminating the global illicit cigarette trade would increase tax revenue and save lives. Paris: International Union Against Tuberculosis and Lung Disease.

Joost, K. (2010) Restrictions proposed to alcohol ads, sales. Baltic Reports: Daily News from the Baltic States [online journal] <http://balticreports.com/2010/01/18/restrictions-proposed-on-alcohol-ads-sales/> (accessed 18 July 2013).

Karachaliou, K., Kontogeorgiou, K., Kitsos, G., et al. (2005) The situation of alcohol use and abuse in Greece. Trastornos Adictivos **7**: 69–79.

Karlsson T., and Österberg, E. (2002) Denmark, in E. Österberg, T. Karlsson (eds), Alcohol policies in EU member states and Norway. A collection of country reports. Helsinki: STAKES, pp. 120–139.

Karlsson, T., and Österberg, E. (2009) Alcohol affordability and cross-border trade in alcohol. Östersund: Swedish National Institute of Public Health.

Karlsson, T., Lindeman, M., and Österberg, E. (2012) Does alcohol policy make any difference? Scales and consumption, in P. Anderson, F. Braddick, J. Reynolds, and A. Gual (eds), Alcohol policy in Europe: Evidence from AMPHORA. The AMPHORA project, available from <http://amphoraproject.net/view.php?id_cont=45>.

Kickert, W., Klijn, E. H., and Koppenjan, J. (1997) Managing complex networks: strategies for the public sector. London: Sage Publications.

Kitschelt, H., Lange, P., Marks, G., et al. (1999) Convergence and divergence in advanced capitalist democracies, in H. Kitschelt, P. Lange, G. Marks, and J. D. Stephens (eds), Continuity and change in contemporary capitalism. New York: Cambridge University Press, pp. 427–460.

Koppenjan, J. and Klijn, EH. (2004) Managing Uncertainties in Networks. Abingdon: Routledge.

Kühlhorn, E., Hibell, B., Larsson, S., et al. (2000) Alcohol consumption in Sweden in the 1990s. Stockholm: Elanders Gotab.

Lachenmeier, D. W., Rehm, J., and Gmel, G. (2007) Surrogate alcohol: what do we know and where do we go?. Alcoholism: Clinical and Experimental Research **31**: 1613–1624.

Laslett, A. M., Catalano, P., Chikritzhs, P., et al. (2010) The range and magnitude of alcohol's harm to others. Fitzroy, Victoria: AER Centre for Alcohol Policy Research, Turning Point Alcohol and Drug Centre, Eastern Health.

Latvia—EMCDDA Country Overview (2011) [website] <http://www.emcdda.europa.eu/publications/country-overviews/lv> (accessed 18 July 2013).

Leibfried, S. (1992) Towards a European welfare state? On integrating poverty regimes into the European Community, in Z. Ferge, and J. E. Kolberg (eds), Social policy in a changing Europe. Frankfurt: Campus Verlag, pp. 133–156.

Leifman, H. (2001) Estimations of unrecorded alcohol consumption levels and trends in 14 European countries, Nordisk alkohol & narkotikatidskrift, Nordic Studies on Alcohol and Drugs, **18** (English Supplement), pp. 54–70.

Lemmens, P. H. (2000) Unrecorded alcohol consumption in the Netherlands: legal, semi-legal and illegal production and trade in alcoholic beverages. Contemporary Drug Problems **27**: 301–313.

Lenton, S., and Single, E. (2004) The definition of harm reduction. Drug and Alcohol Review **17**: 213–240.

Levi, M. (1997) A model, a method and a map: Rational choice in comparative and historical analysis, in M. I. Lichbach, and A. S. Zuckerman (eds), Comparative politics: rationality, culture and structure. Cambridge: Cambridge University Press, pp. 19–41.

Lewy, J. (2008) The drug policy of the Third Reich. Social History of Alcohol and Drugs **22**: 144–167.

Lim, S. S., Vos, T., Flaxman, A. D., et al. (2012) A comparative risk assessment of burden of disease and injury attributable to 67 risk factors and risk factor clusters in 21 regions, 1990–2010: a systematic analysis for the Global Burden of Disease Study 2010. Lancet **380**: 2224–2260.

Lipovestky, G. (2008) La felicidad paradójica. Barcelona: Anagrama.

Lithuania—EMCDDA Country Overview (2011) [website] <http://www.emcdda.europa.eu/publications/country-overviews/lt> (accessed 18 July 2013).

The Lithuania Tribune (2010) World drugs report 2010: Estonia in 2nd place. The Lithuania Tribune: News and Views from Lithuania [online journal], <http://www.lithuaniatribune.com/2010/06/30/world-drugs-report-2010-estonia-in-2nd-place> (accessed 18 July 2013).

Loi Évin (1991) Loi no 91–32 du 10 janvier 1991 relative à la lutte contre le tabagisme et l'alcoolisme.

Lozano, J. M., Albareda, L., Ysa, T., et al. (2006) Governments and corporate social responsibility: Public policies beyond regulation and voluntary compliance. Basingstoke: Palgrave.

Luxembourg—EMCDDA Country Overview (2011) [website] <http://www.emcdda. europa.eu/publications/country-overviews/lu> (accessed 18 July 2013).

Mäkelä, K. (1979) Unrecorded consumption of alcohol in Finland, 1950–1975. Reports from the Social Research Institute of Alcohol Studies 126. Helsinki: Social Research Institute of Alcohol Studies.

Mäkelä, P. et al. (2001) Episodic heavy drinking in four Nordic countries: A comparative survey. Addiction **96**: 1575–1588.

Mäkelä, P., Fonager, K., Hibell, B., et al. (1999) Drinking habits in the Nordic countries. SIFA, Rapport 2/1999. Oslo: SIFA.

Malczewski, A. (2011) Poland new development: Trends and in-depth information on selected issues draft. 2011 National Report (2010 data) to the EMCDDA by the Reitox Polish Reitox Focal Point.

Malinowska-Sempruch, K. (2012) The end of marijuana prohibition: Project Syndicate [online journal], <http://www.project-syndicate.org/commentary/legalizing-marijuana-in-washington-and-colorado-by-kasia-malinowska-sempruch> (accessed 18 July 2013).

Malta—EMCDDA Country Overview (2011) [website] <http://www.emcdda.europa.eu/ publications/country-overviews/mt> (accessed 18 July 2013).

Mamudu, H. M., and Studlar, D. T. (2009) Multilevel governance and shared sovereignty: European Union, member states, and the FCTC. Governance **22**: 73–97.

Marlise, S. (2002) Elections to proceed in the Netherlands, despite killing. New York Times [online journal] <http://www.nytimes.com/2002/05/08/world/elections-to-proceed-in-the-netherlands-despite-killing.html> (accessed 18 July 2013).

Martí, O. (1998) Todo lo que quisiste saber sobre la dependencia de las drogas y nunca te atreviste a preguntar. Hondarribia: Argitaletxe Hiru.

Martínez Oró, D. P., Pallarés, J., Barruti, M., et al. (2010) Observatori de nous consums de drogues en l'àmbit juvenil. Informe 2009. Barcelona: Fundació IGenus.

Megías, I. (2009) El concepto de normalidad en el contexto de los riesgos asociados a los y las jóvenes y la gestión de oportunidades. Revista Juventud **82**: 47–65.

Mendoza, X., Vernis, A. (2008) The changing role of governments and the emergence of the relational state. Corporate Governance **8**: 389–396.

Møller, L. (2002) Legal restrictions resulted in a reduction of alcohol consumption among young people in Denmark, in R. Room (ed.), The effects of Nordic alcohol policies: Analyses of changes in control systems. Helsinki: Nordic Council for Alcohol and Drug Research, pp. 155–166.

Moser, J. (1992) Alcohol problems, policies and programmes in Europe. Copenhagen: WHO Regional Office for Europe.

Mravčík, V., Pešek, R., Horáková, M., et al. (2010) Annual report: The Czech Republic—2009 drug situation. Prague: Úřad vlády České republiky.

Netherlands—EMCDDA Country Overview (2011) [website] <http://www.emcdda. europa.eu/publications/country-overviews/nl> (accessed 18 July 2013).

Nieva, P., Baulenas, G., and Borràs, T. (1995) Centros de encuentro y acogida. Madrid: PNSD.

Nohlen, D. and Stöver, P. (2010) Elections in Europe: A data handbook. Nomos.

NordAN (2011) Copenhagen is heading toward legalizing cannabis. NordAN 49/2011.

Nordlund, S. (1985) Norwegian drinking habits, description based on official statistics and survey-data, in O. Arner, R. Hauge, and O. J. Skog (eds), Alcohol in Norway. Oslo: Universitetsforlaget, pp. 46–70.

Nordlund, S. (1992) Methods and problems in estimating the amount of alcohol consumption. SIFA, Rapport 3/1992. Oslo: SIFA.

Norström, T. (1998) Estimating changes in unrecorded alcohol consumption in Norway using indicators of harm. Addiction **93**: 1531–1538.

Norway—EMCDDA Country Overview (2011) [website] <http://www.emcdda.europa.eu/publications/country-overviews/no> (accessed 18 July 2013).

Norwegian Ministry of Health and Care Services (2007) Norwegian national action plan on alcohol and drugs 2007–2010.

Nye, J. (2004) Soft power: The means to success in world politics. New York: Public Affairs.

OECD (2011a) How's life? Measuring well-being. Paris: OECD Publishing.

OECD (2011b) Compendium of OECD well-being indicators. Paris: OECD Better Life Initiative.

OECD (2011c) [website] <http://www.oecdbetterlifeindex.org> (accessed 18 July 2013).

O'Hare, P. A. (1995) La reducción de daños relacionados con las drogas. Barcelona: Grup IGIA.

OKANA (2012) [website] <http://www.okana.gr/2012-04-03-07-49-40/item/253> (accessed 18 July 2013).

Oleaque, J. M. (2004) En éxtasi. Barcelona: Ara llibres.

Origer, A. (2009) Grand Duchy of Luxembourg. New developments, trends and in-depth information on selected issues. 2009 National Report (2008 data) to the EMCDDA by the Reitox National Focal Point. Centre de Reserche Public & EMCDDA.

Österberg, E. (2000) Unrecorded alcohol consumption in Finland in the 1990s. Contemporary Drug Problems **27**: 271–299.

Österberg, E. and Karlsson, T. (2002) Alcohol policies in EU member states and Norway: A collection of country reports. Helsinki: STAKES.

Österberg, E. and Pehkonen, J. (1996) Travellers' imports of alcoholic beverages into Finland before and after EU. Nordisk Alkoholtidskrift/Nordic Alcohol Studies 13 (English suppl.): 22–32.

O'Toole, L. J. (1997) Treating networks seriously: Practical and research-based agendas in public administration. Public Administration Review **57**: 45–52.

Pallarés, J. (1995) La dolça punxada de l'escorpí. Lleida: Pagès Editors.

Pallarés, J., Díaz, A., Barruti, M., et al. (2006) Observatori de nous consums de drogues en l'àmbit juvenil. Metodologia i Informe evolutiu 1999–2005. Barcelona: Departament de Salut Generalitat de Catalunya.

Paskin, B. (2013) UK government scraps minimum pricing plans. The Spirits Business [online journal] <http://www.thespiritsbusiness.com/2013/07/uk-government-scraps-minimum-pricing-plans/> (accessed 22 November 2013).

Pavarini, M. (1983) Control y dominación. Teorías criminológicas burguesas y proyecto hegemónico. México DF: Siglo XXI.

Peek, J. (1994) International police cooperation within justified political and judicial frameworks: Five theses on TREVI, in J. Monar, and R. Morgan (eds), The third pillar of the European Union. Brussels: European Interuniversity Press, pp. 201–207.

Poland—EMCDDA Country Overview (2011) [website] <http://www.emcdda.europa.eu/publications/country-overviews/pl> (accessed 18 July 2013).

Polish Government (2011) Polish national programme for counteracting drug addiction 2011–2016.

Pollit, C. and Bouckaert, G. (2009) Continuity and Change in Public Policy and Management. Cheltenham: Edward Elgar Publishing.

Pollit, C. and Bouckaert, G. (2011) Public Management Reform. A Comparative Analysis: New Public Management, Governance, and the Neo-Weberian State. Oxford: Oxford University Press.

Popova, S., Rehm, J., Patra, J., et al. (2007) Comparing alcohol consumption in central and Eastern Europe to other European countries. Alcohol and Alcoholism **42**: 465–473.

Portugal—EMCDDA Country Overview (2011) [website] <http://www.emcdda.europa.eu/publications/country-overviews/pt> (accessed 18 July 2013).

Portugal—EMCDDA Legal Profile (2011) [website] <http://www.emcdda.europa.eu/html.cfm/index5174EN.html?pluginMethod=eldd.countryprofiles&country=PT> (accessed 18 July 2013).

Portugal—EMCDDA Policy Profile (2011) Drug policy profile. Luxembourg: Publications Office of the European Union.

Publico (2011) Descriminalização da droga facilitou toxicodependentes a irem para tratamento. Publico [online journal] <http://www.publico.pt/n1496129> (accessed 18 July 2013).

Quigley, E., Costa-Storti, C. C., and Hughes, B. (2013) Illicit drugs in Europe: Supply, demand and public policies. Presentation at EMCDDA European Summer School.

Rabinovich, L., Brutscher, P. B., de Vries, H., et al. (2009) The affordability of alcoholic beverages in the European Union: Understanding the link between alcohol affordability, consumption and harms. RAND Europe Technical Report.

Ramstedt, M. (2006) What drug policies cost: Estimating drug policy expenditures in Sweden, 2002: Work in progress. Addiction **101**: 330–338.

RAND Europe (2012) [website] <http://www.rand.org/randeurope/about.html> (accessed 18 July 2013).

Rehm, J. (2012) What alcohol can do to European societies, in P. Anderson, F. Braddick, J. Reynolds, et al. (eds), Alcohol policy in Europe: Evidence from AMPHORA. The AMPHORA project, available online: <http://amphoraproject.net/view.php?id_cont=45> (accessed 18 July 2013).

Rehm, J., Marmet, S., Anderson, P. et al. (2013) Defining substance use disorders: do we really need more than heavy use? Alcohol and Alcoholism **48**: 633–640.

Rehm, J., Shield, K., Rehm, M., et al. (2012) Alcohol consumption, alcohol dependence, and attributable burden of diseasen in Europe: potential gains from effective interventions for alcohol dependence. Toronto: Center for Addiction and Mental Health.

Reinås, K. T. (1991) The sources of alcohol: The total alcohol consumption in Norway. Oslo: Rusmiddeldirektoratet.

Retailers against smuggling (2012) [website] <http://www.retailersagainstsmuggling.ie> (accessed 18 July 2013).

Reuter, P., and Trautmann, F. (2009) A report on global illicit drugs markets 1998–2007. Full Report. European Commission, RAND Europe, Trimbos Institute.

Rhodes, T. and Hedrich, D. (2010) Harm reduction: Evidence, impacts and challenges. EMCDDA Monographs: 10. Luxembourg: Publications Office of the European Union.

Rittel, H. and Webber, M. (1973) Dilemmas in a general theory of planning. Policy Sciences, **4**: 155–169.

Ritter, A. (2009) How do drug policy makers access research evidence? International Journal of Drug Policy **20**: 70–75.

Ritter, A. (2010) Illicit drugs policy through the lens of regulation. International Journal of Drug Policy **21**: 265–270.

Ritter, A. and Bammer, G. (2010) Models of policy making and their relevance for drug research. Drug and Alcohol Review **29**: 352–357.

Ritter, A. and Lancaster, K. (2012) Measuring research influence on drug policy: A case example of two epidemiological monitoring systems. International Journal of Drug Policy **24**: 30–37.

Ritter, K. (2007) Governing Center Party edges opposition in Finnish election. Independent. March 19.

Romaní, O. (1997) Etnografía y drogas. Discursos y prácticas. Nueva Antropologia XVI **52**: 39–66.

Romaní, O. (1999) Las drogas. Sueños y Razones. Barcelona: Ariel.

Romaní, O. (2008) Políticas de drogas: prevención, participación, y reducción del daño. Salud Colectiva **4**: 301–318.

Romaní, O. (2009) Criticando estereotipos. Jóvenes, drogas y riesgos. Congreso Hablemos de Drogas. Barcelona 3–5 Juny de 2005: FAD i Fundació La Caixa.

Romaní, O. and Comelles, J. M. (1991) Les condictions liées à l'usage des psychotropes dans les societés contemporaines: automédication et dépendance. Psychoytopes **10**: 39–57.

Romaní, O., Espinal, N., and Rovira, J. M. (1989) Presa de contacte amb els drogodependents d'alt risc. Barcelona: Institut Municipal de Salut.

Romania—EMCDDA Country Overview (2011) [website] <http://www.emcdda.europa.eu/publications/country overviews/ro> (accessed 18 July 2013).

Room, R. (1992) The impossible dream? Routes to reducing alcohol problems in a temperance culture. Journal of Substance Abuse **4**: 91–106.

Room, R., Jernigan, D., Marlatt, B. C., et al. (2002) Alcohol in developing societies: A public health approach. Helsinki: Finnish Foundation for Alcohol Studies.

Room, R. and Mäkelä, K. (2000) Typologies of the cultural position of drinking. Journal of Studies on Alcohol **61**: 475–483.

Rosenquist, J. N., Murabito, J., Fowler, J. H., et al. (2010) The spread of alcohol consumption behaviour in a large social network. Annals of Internal Medicine **152**: 426–433.

Rosenqvist, P. and Kurube, N. (1992) Dissolving the Swedish alcohol-treatment system, in H. Klingemann, J. P. Takala, and G. Hunt (eds), Cure, care, or control: Alcoholism treatment in sixteen countries, Albany: State University of New York Press, pp. 65–86.

Rosmarin, A. and Eastwood, N. (2012) A quiet revolution: Drug decriminalisation policies in practice across the globe, Release: Drugs, The Law & Human Rights.

Ruchansky, E. (2012) El camino portugués. Página 12 [online journal] <http://www.pagina12.com.ar/diario/sociedad/3-196054-2012-06-10.html> (accessed 18 July 2013).

Savutonsuomi (2012) [website] <http://www.savutonsuomi.fi/en.php> (accessed 18 July 2013).

Schedler, K. and Proeller, I. (2010) Outcome-Oriented Public Management. A Responsibility-Based Approach to the New Public Management. Charlotte: IAP-Information Age Publishing.

Sevcenko, M. (2010) Prague: the new Amsterdam? Global Post: America's World New Site [online journal], <http://www.globalpost.com/dispatch/czech-republic/101127/marijuana-laws> (accessed 18 July 2013).

Simpura, J. and Karlsson, T. (2001) Trends in drinking patterns in fifteen European countries, 1950–2000. A collection of country reports. Helsinki: STAKES.

Slovakia—EMCDDA Country Overview (2011) [website] <http://www.emcdda.europa.eu/publications/country-overviews/sk> (accessed 18 July 2013).

Slovenia EMCDDA Country Overview (2011) [website] <http://www.emcdda.europa.eu/publications/country-overviews/si> (accessed 18 July 2013).

Slovenian Government (2004) Resolution on the national programme in the field of drugs 2004–2009.

Spain—EMCDDA Country Overview (2011) [website] <http://www.emcdda.europa.eu/publications/country-overviews/es> (accessed 18 July 2013).

Spanish Ministry of Health and Social Affairs (2009) Spanish drug action plan 2009–2012

Spear, B. (1994) The early years of the Bristish system in practice, in J. Strang and M. Gossop (eds), Heroin addicition and drug policy: The British system. Oxford: Oxford University Press, pp. 3–28.

Spode, H. (1993) Die Macht der Trunkenheit: Kultur- und Sozialgeschichte des Alkohols in Deutschland Opladen. Leverkusen: Verlag Leske & Budrich.

STAKES (2001) Yearbook of alcohol and drug statistics 1997–2001. Helsinki, STAKES.

Steber, D. and Dreifuss, R. (2012) Suiza. A: Regulando las Guerras Contra las Drogas. Londres: Ideas.

Stenius, K. (1999) Private and public in the Swedish treatment system. Division of tasks, cooperation and steering during the 1990s. Lund: Arkiv förlag.

Stewart-Clark, J. (1987) Committee of inquiry into the drugs problem in the Member States of the Community: Report on the results of the Enquiry. European Parliament.

Stiglitz, J. E., Sen, A., and Fitoussi, J. P. (2009) Report by the Commission on the Measurement of Economic Performance and Social Progress [online] <http://www.stiglitz-sen-fitoussi.fr/documents/rapport_anglais.pdf> (accessed 18 July 2013).

Stoker, G. (1998) Governance as theory: five propositions. International Social Science Journal, **50**: 17–28.

Stratégie et plan d'action gouvernementaux 2010-2014 en matière de lutte contre les drogues et les addictions (2010) Ministère de Santé - Direction de la Santé, Cellule de Coordination Drogues, Le Gouvernement du Grand-Duché de Luxembourg.

Sullivan, R. J. and Hagen, E. H. (2002) Psychotropic substance-seeking: evolutionary pathology or adaptation? Addiction **97**: 389–400.

Summaries of EU legislation (Community Tobacco Fund) (2012) [website] <http://europa.eu/legislation_summaries/public_health/health_determinants_lifestyle/c11577_en.htm> (accessed 18 July 2013).

Sustainable Governance Indicators (2011) [website] <http://www.sgi-network.org/> (accessed 18 July 2013).

Sweden—EMCDDA Country Overview (2011) [website] <http://www.emcdda.europa.eu/publications/country-overviews/se> (accessed 18 July 2013).

Swedish Ministry of Health and Social Affairs (2011) A cohesive strategy for alcohol, narcotic drugs, doping and tobacco (ANDT) policy. Regeringskansliet, Ministry of Health and Social Affairs, Sweden.

Swedish National Institute of Public Health (website) <http://www.fhi.se/encoordinates> (accessed 18 July 2013).

Szalavitz, M. (2009) Drugs in Portugal: Did decriminalization work? Time: Science & Space [online journal] <http://www.time.com/time/health/article/0,8599,1893946,00.html> (accessed 18 July 2013).

Theodoropoulos, M. (2012) No more time to waste, prohibition has failed. ENCOD Bulletin on Drug Policies in Europe.

Tiessen, J., Hunt, P., Celia, C., et al. (2010) Assessing the impacts of revising the tobacco products directive: Study to support a DG SANCO Impact Assessment. Final report. RAND Europe.

Transparency International—Corruption Perception Index [website] (2011) <http://cpi. transparency.org/cpi2012/> (accessed 18 July 2013).

Trautmann, F. (2013) Key trends of the illicit drugs market and drug policy in the EU: What do experts anticipate for the coming years?, in F. Trautmann, B. Kilmer, and P. Turnbull (eds), Further insights into aspects of the EU illicit drugs market. Luxembourg: Publications Office of the European Union, pp. 447–501.

Trigueiros, F., Vitória, P. and Dias, L. (2010) Rather treat than punish: The Portuguese decriminalization model. Expert forum on criminal justice: national experiences with quasi-coerced treatment of drug dependent offenders, Pompidou Group of the Council of Europe, Strasbourg.

Trolldal, B. (2001) Alcohol sales figures in 15 European countries: corrected for consumption abroad and tax-free purchases. Nordic Studies on Alcohol and Drugs **18**: 71–81.

Ugland, T. (2011) Alcohol on the European Union's political agenda: Getting off the policy roller-coaster? Norwegian Institute for Alcohol and Drug Research. SIRUS Report 1/2011.

UK Drug Strategy (2010) Reducing demand, restricting supply, building recovery: Supporting people to live a drug free life. London: H.M. Government.

United Kingdom—EMCDDA Country Overview (2011) [website] <http://www.emcdda. europa.eu/publications/country-overviews/uk> (accessed 18 July 2013).

United Kingdom Home Office (2012) [website] <http://www.homeoffice.gov.uk/drugs/ alcohol/alcohol-pricing/> (accessed 18 July 2013).

United Nations (1961) Single Convention on Narcotic Drugs. United Nations Conventions.

United Nations (1971a) Convention on Psychotropic Substances. United Nations Conventions.

United Nations (1971b) Single Convention on Narcotic Drugs, 1961. As amended by the 1972 Protocol amending the Single Convention on Narcotic Drugs. United Nations Conventions.

United Nations (1988) Convention against illicit traffic in narcotic drugs and psychotropic substances. United Nations Conventions.

United Nations (2004a) Convention against Corruption. United Nations Conventions.

United Nations (2004b) UN Convention against Transnational organized crime. United Nations Conventions. Full text: <http://www.unodc.org/unodc/en/treaties/ CTOC/#Fulltext> (accessed 18 July 2013).

United Nations (2007) UN Convention Committee on the Rights of the Child (2007) CRC/C/PRT/3-4: Committee on the Rights of the Child Consideration of the reports submitted by States parties under article 44 of the Convention Third and fourth periodic reports of States parties due in 2007 Portugal.

United Nations Treaty Collection Database [website] <treaties.un.org/pages/View-Details.aspx?src=TREATY&mtdsg_no=IX-4&chapter=9&lang=en> (accessed 18 July 2013).

UNODC (2007) Sweden's Successful Drug Policy: A Review of the Evidence.

UNODC (2010) World drug report. Vienna: United Nations Publications.

UNODC (2011a) Global Afghan opiate trade: A threat assessment. Vienna: United Nations Publications.

UNODC (2011b) World Drug Report. New York: United Nations Publications.

UNODC and Afghanistan Ministry of Counter Narcotics (2011a) Afghanistan opium survey 2011. Afghanistan Ministry of Counter-Narcotics, UNODC-Kabul and UNODC-Vienna.

UNODC and Afghanistan Ministry of Counter Narcotics (2011b) Afghanistan cannabis survey 2010. Afghanistan Ministry of Counter-Narcotics, UNODC-Kabul and UNODC-Vienna.

Usó Arnal, J. C. (1996) Drogas y cultura de masas. España 1855-1995. Madrid: Taurus.

Usó Arnal, J. C. (2010) Prevención de salón en España durante la dictadura de Primo de Rivera. La Asociación contra la Toxicomanía (1926–1931). Health and Addictions/Salud y Drogas 10: 51–78.

Van Dam, T. (2007) International drug user movement. Adviesbureau Theo van Dam: Avies vanuit client perspectief [online] <http://www.lsd.nl/Adviesbureau/Diensten/drug_user_movement.html> (accessed 18 July 2013).

Van Solinge, T. B. (1999) Dutch drug policy in a European context. Journal of Drug Issues 29: 511–528.

Van Solinge, T. B. (2002) Drugs and decision-making in the European Union. Journal of Cognitive Liberties 3: 63–100.

Vergne, J. P. and Duran, R. (2010) Path dependence and path creation: Alternative Theoretical and methodological perspectives on strategy, innovation and entrepreneurship. Journal of Management Studies 47: 733–735.

WHO (2003) Framework Convention on Tobacco Control. World Health Organization Conventions.

WHO (2004) Global status report on alcohol and health. Geneva: World Health Organization.

WHO (2005a) Global information system on alcohol and health: levels of consumption [website] <http://apps.who.int/gho/data/node.main> (accessed 18 July 2013).

WHO (2005b) Levels of consumption: Recorded adult per capita consumption, from 1961, total by country [website] <http://apps.who.int/gho/data/node.main.A1025?lang=en?showonly=GISAH> (accessed 18 July 2013).

WHO (2005c) Levels of Consumption: Unrecorded adult per capita consumption by country [website] <http://apps.who.int/gho/data/node.main.A1034?lang=en> (accessed 18 July 2013).

WHO (2010) International classification of diseases—10. Geneva: WHO.

WHO (2011a) Global status report on alcohol and health. Switzerland: WHO.

WHO (2011b) Governance for health in the 21st century: A study conducted for the WHO Regional Office for Europe. Geneva: WHO.

WHO (2013) Status report on alcohol and health in 35 European countries 2013. Geneva: WHO.

Wil, A. and Gelissen, J. (2002) Three worlds of welfare capitalism or more? A state-of-the-art report. Journal of European Social Policy **12**: 137–158.

Williams I., Kemp, S., Coello, J., et al. (2012) A beginner's guide to carbon footprinting. Carbon Management **3**: 55–67.

World Drink Trends (2002) Henley-on-Thames, United Kingdom, Productschap voor Gedistilleerde Dranken and World Advertising Research Center Ltd.

World Economic Forum and WHO (2011) From burden to 'best buys': Reducing the economic impact of non-communicable diseases in low- and middle-income countries. Geneva: World Economic Forum.

World Values Survey (2012) [website] <http://www.worldvaluessurvey.org> (accessed 18 July 2013).

Ysa, T., Sierra, V., and Esteve, M. (2014) Determinants of network outcomes: The impact of managerial strategies. Public Administration. Forthcoming.

Zatonski, W., Manczuk M., and Sulkowska, U. (2008) Closing the health gap in the European Union. Warsaw, Cancer Epidemiology and Prevention Division, The Maria Sklodowska-Curie Memorial Cancer Centre and Institute of Oncology.

Zemblicka, A. (2011) Tobacco smuggling in the Baltic states increases. Bright: Organising media against organised crime, March 28 [online] <http://www.flarenetwork.org/report/top_news_100615/article/tobacco_smuggling_in_the_baltic_states_increases.htm> (accessed 18 July 2013).

Zeugles, D. W. (2006) International trade agreements challenge tobacco and alcohol control policies. Drug and Alcohol Review **25**: 567–579.

Index

A

addiction
  concepts 2–3
  growing global concern 1–3
ad hoc coordinating bodies 122, 141, 160
  model 1 countries 50, 53–4, 57, 58–9, 63, 66–7
  model 2 countries 74, 76, 78, 80, 82–3, 86
  model 3 countries 92, 96
  model 4 countries 107, 108, 109–10, 112, 116
advertising, alcohol and tobacco 31, 81
Advisory Council on the Misuse of Drugs (ACMD), UK 83
Afghanistan 39
AIDS *see* HIV/AIDS
Albareda, A. xv
alcohol
  deaths related to 2, 41, 104
  geopolitics 41
  minimum unit pricing 84
alcohol consumption
  European countries 70
  model 1 countries 53, 56, 65–6
  model 2 countries 69–70, 80
  model 4 countries 103–4
  Slovenia 99
  variables 151–2
alcohol industry 37
alcohol policy and control
  classification 14, 16, 17
  EU 31, 32, 35–6, 41
  model 1 countries 57
  model 2 countries 76, 78, 80, 81, 82
  model 3 countries 93, 98, 99
  model 4 countries 104–5, 107, 108, 110, 112, 115
  role of international organizations 42
  stakeholder involvement 37–8
alcohol policy scale 158
alcohol policy scales 16, 139–40
  European countries 73
  model 1 countries 57, 58, 65
  model 2 countries 76, 78, 80, 86
  model 3 countries 90, 91, 93, 95
  model 4 countries 111, 116
alco-locks 98
ALICE RAP project 26
Alko Inc., Finland 78
Amsterdam Treaty (1999) 32, 34

Anderson, P. v–viii
Anglo-Saxon countries 69, 70, 86–7
assistentialism 4
Austria 89, 92–4, 162–3

B

Balkan Route, drug trafficking 39, 109, 111, 115
Baltic states 104–5, 117
Belgium 52–4, 164–5
Bertelsmann Stiftung indicators 10
best practices, EMCDDA, top-rated 140, 160
  model 1 countries 52, 54, 58, 60, 64, 66, 68
  model 2 countries 84, 87
  model 3 countries 91
Better Life Initiative, OECD 10, 12–13, 145
Brewers of Europe (BoE) 37
Bulgaria 89, 94–6, 166–7
  as heroin gateway 39, 94, 95
Bundesdrogenforum (Federal Drug Forum, FDF), Austria 93–4
businesses, involvement in decision-making 122, 123, 141

C

cannabis
  consumption 49, 153–4
  geopolitics 39–40
  model 1 countries 53, 55, 61, 62, 65
  model 2 countries 70–1
  policy trends 6
Carrión, M. xv
Catholic Europe group 89
CELAD (European Committee to Combat Drugs) 31, 44
Central and Eastern European countries (CEECs) 54–5, 103–17
Civil Society Forum on Drugs (CSF), European 37, 123
civil society groups 36–8, 123
classification, public policies and programmes 11–17, 26
classification (drug) determines penalties variable 139
cluster analysis 22–4
  codified variables 143–4
  operationalization of variables 139–42
  variables and their definitions 145–61
cocaine 4, 5, 27

Colom, J. xv
Comité Européen des Entreprises Vins
    (CEEV) 37
Commission for the Dissuasion of Drug
    Abuse, Portugal 63
Commission for the National Strategy to Fight
    against Drugs, Portugal 62
Commission on Narcotic Drugs (CND) 34
Committee of Permanent Representatives
    (COREPER) 32
Community Action Programme on the
    Prevention of Drug Dependence
    (1996–2000) 32
comprehensive policy approach 21, 22, 122
Confederation of European Community
    Cigarette Manufacturers (CECCM) 37
consumerist model of drugs 3, 4
contextual indicators 9–11, 12–13
Continental countries 67, 89, 127
contingent comparative approach 126–7
Cooney Report (1992) 31
cooperation, international
    EU and other countries/regions 43
    between EU member states 42–3
Corruption Perception Index 12–13, 148
country tables 18, 162–217
    template 134–8
crime, organized 30, 31
criminal penalties
    model 1 countries 53, 56–7, 63
    model 2 countries 72–4, 80, 81
    model 3 countries 91, 93, 95, 96, 97, 99
    model 4 countries 106, 109, 111, 115
    see also decriminalization of drug use
Cyprus 89, 96–7, 168–9
Cyprus Anti-Drugs Council (CAC) 96
Czech Republic 41, 54–6, 170–1

D
deaths, addiction-related 1–2, 108
decentralized policy-making and
    implementation 49, 142, 161
decriminalization of drug use 6, 139
    model 1 countries 47, 48, 51, 55, 61–2, 65
    model 2 countries 72, 76, 77
    model 3 countries 91, 93
    model 4 countries 104, 112, 113
    see also criminal penalties
demand reduction 17
    EU policies 32, 34–5
    model 3 countries 91
Denmark 89, 97–8, 172–3
dependence 2
drug trafficking 30, 31
    model 2 countries 79–80
    model 3 countries 93
    Portugal 63
    routes into EU 39, 109, 111, 112, 115

drug use
    EU policies 27–35
    geopolitics 38–40
    historical aspects 3–6
Dublin Group 36

E
economic crisis 81, 110, 128–9
EMCDDA see European Monitoring Centre
    for Drugs and Drug Addiction
EmPeCemos programme 66
Esping-Andersen welfare state regimes 9–10,
    12–13, 126–7
Estonia 104–5, 107–8, 174–5
Europe Against Drugs (EURAD) 38
European Alcohol and Health Forum 38, 123
European Alcohol Policy Alliance
    (Eurocare) 37, 38
European Cigar Manufacturers Association
    (ECMA) 37
European Committee to Combat Drugs
    (CELAD) 31, 44
European Confederation of Tobacco Retailers
    (ECTR) 37
European Directives
    alcohol excise duty 32
    tobacco control 32–4, 35, 40
European Economic Community (EEC)
    27–31
European Forum for Responsible Drinking
    (EFRD) 37
European Monitoring Centre for Drugs and
    Drug Addiction (EMCDDA) 31
    top-rated best practices see best practices,
        EMCDDA, top-rated
European Plan to Combat Drugs 31
European Public Health Alliance (EPHA)
    37–8
European Smoking Tobacco Association
    (ESTA) 37
European Union (EU) policy 18, 27–45, 123,
    128
    achievements 42–3
    common features of member states'
        policies 42–3
    historical aspects 27–36
    models and visions for governance of
        addictions 129
    models of governance of addictions see
        models of governance of addictions
    role of international organizations 41–2
    stakeholder involvement 36–8
    conclusions 44–5
Europol Drugs Unit (EDU) 31
evidence-based approaches 20, 121
    model 2 countries 71, 74, 87
excise duty, alcohol 32
experts, interviews with 17–18, 131–3

F

family motivational intervention 60
Fantastyczne Mozliwosci programme 91
Federal Drug Commissioner, Germany 51
Federal Drug Coordination Office (FDCO),
    Austria 93–4
Federal Drug Forum (FDF;
    Bundesdrogenforum), Austria 93–4
Finland 77–9, 176–7
    influence on EU policies 32
    substance consumption 69, 71
    tobacco-free by 2040 initiative 78, 79
Framework Convention on Tobacco Control
    (FCTC), WHO 35, 41–2, 155
France 69, 79–81, 178–9

G

GDP per capita 149
General Drugs Policy Cell, Belgium 53–4
Geneva Convention (1936) 4
geopolitics of addictive substances 38–41
Germany 50–2, 180–1
GINI index 150
governance
    concept 7
    indicators, sustainable 10, 12–13
governance of addictions 6–7
    European models and visions 129
    framework and trends 120–3
    model for analysis 19, 20, 119–20
    models *see* models of governance
        of addictions
    research methodology 9–26
Gower's similarity measure 22
Greece 103, 104, 109–10, 182–3
    as heroin gateway 39, 109
Grow Up Playing programme 64

H

Hague International Opium Convention, The
    (1912) 1
harm reduction
    EU member states' policies 42–3
    EU policies 34–5
    historical context 5, 6
    model 1 countries 48, 58
    model 2 countries 72–4, 76, 80, 84, 86
    model 3 countries 92, 93, 96, 97
    model 4 countries 106, 108, 112, 113–14,
        116
health-oriented policies 34–5, 44, 121
'heavy use over time' 3
hepatitis B 5
heroin
    gateways to Europe 39, 94, 95, 109, 112
    geopolitics 38–9
    policy trends 6

heroin (opiate) consumption 49
    Estonia 108
    Greece 110
    historical aspects 4–5, 27
    model 2 countries 71
    variables 154
historical aspects
    EU addictions policy 27–36
    substance use 3–6
HIV/AIDS 5, 27, 65, 108, 110
Horizontal Drugs Group (HDG) 32, 35
Hungary 110–11, 184–5

I

illicit substances
    classification of public policies 15, 17
    EU policies 27–31
    geopolitics 38–40
    model 1 approaches 47–8, 68
    model 2 approaches 72–4
    tackled jointly with legal substances 140
    trendsetters in *see* model 1
inequality, high levels 83, 86, 89
information
    gathering 11–17
    triangulating sources of 17–18
Inglehart World Values Survey 11, 12–13,
    147–8
injection rooms 139, 158
    model 1 countries 48, 51, 65, 68
    model 2 countries 72, 86
    model 3 countries 91–2
Institute on Drugs and Drug Addiction (IDT),
    Portugal 63, 64
Inter-ministerial Commission on Drugs
    (ICDL), Luxembourg 58–9
Inter-ministerial Mission for the Fight against
    Drugs and Drug Addiction (MILDT) 80
International Narcotics Control Board
    (INCB) 42
international organizations 41–2
interviews, with experts 17–18, 131–3
Ireland 72, 81–3, 186–7
    substance consumption 69, 70
Italy 56–8, 188–9

J

Junkie Unions, the Netherlands 5

K

Kasse200 programme 52
Konsumentverket, Sweden 76

L

Länder, Germany 51, 52
Latvia 104–5, 111–13, 190–1
law enforcement approach 30, 32, 44

legal sanctions *see* criminal penalties
legal substances 139–40
  classification of public policies 14, 16–17
  EU policies 31, 32–4, 35–6
  geopolitics 40–1
  model 1 approaches 48–50, 68
  model 2 approaches 69–70, 74
  regulation model *see* model 2
  tackled jointly with illicit substances 140
Lithuania 104–5, 113–14, 192–3
Loi Évin, France 80, 81
Luxembourg 58–9, 194–5

M
Maastricht Treaty (1993) 31, 44
Malta 103, 104, 114–15, 196–7
management index 10, 146
media coverage, analysis of 17
Mediterranean countries 67, 103, 127
methodology, research 9–26
  challenges and limitations 24–6, 127
  cluster analysis 22–4
  contextual indicators 9–11, 12–13
  information gathering 11–17
  model for analysis 19, 20
  models of governance of addictions 19–22, 25
  triangulating sources of information 17–18
Ministries of Interior or Justice 122
  model 1 countries 58, 60, 62–3, 65
  model 2 countries 83
  model 3 countries 97
  model 4 countries 103, 111, 114, 116
Ministry of Health 121, 139
  model 1 countries 51, 55, 57, 58, 60, 62–3, 64, 65, 67
  model 2 countries 75, 82, 83, 85
  model 3 countries 92, 93–4, 97, 100
  model 4 countries 109, 111
model 1 (trendsetters in illicit substances) 25, 47–68, 121, 123–5
  description 47–50
  key elements 48
  specific countries 50–67
  conclusions 67–8
model 2 (regulation of legal substances) 25, 69–87, 121, 124, 125
  description 69–74
  key elements 72
  specific countries 74–86
  conclusions 86–7
model 3 (transitioning) 25, 89–101, 124, 125
  description 89–90
  key elements 90
  specific countries 90–100
  conclusions 100–1
model 4 (traditional approach) 25, 103–17, 124, 125–6
  description 103–5
  key elements 104

specific countries 105–16
  conclusions 116–17
model for analysis of governance of
  addictions 19, 20, 119–20
models of governance of addictions 19–22, 25, 119–20, 123–6
moral paradigm 3–4
Morocco 39, 65

N
Narcotics Act, 1981 (Germany) 50–1
National Advisory Committee on Drugs, Ireland 83
National Anti-drug Agency (NAA), Romania 116
National Board of Health and Welfare, Swedish 77
National Committee of Anti-Drug Policy, Italy 57
National Council for the Fight Against Drugs, Drug Addiction and the Harmful Use of Alcohol, Portugal 63
National Institute of Public Health, Swedish 76–7
needle and syringe exchange 43, 75, 80, 92, 108
Netherlands, the 59–61, 198–9
  influence on EU policies 35
non-profit organizations 38, 122, 141, 161
  model 1 countries 52, 56, 59
Nordic countries 127
  model 2 69–70, 71, 86–7
  model 3 89
normalization, drug use 5
Norway 69, 85–6, 200–1

O
objectives of national strategy, addiction on 141
OKANA (Organization Against Drugs), Greece 109–10
opiates *see* heroin
Opioid Substitution Treatment (OST) 43
Opiumgesetz (German Opium law) (1929) 50
Opium Law, the Netherlands 59
Organization for Economic Co-operation and Development (OECD), Better Life Initiative 10, 12–13, 145
organized crime 30, 31
Oversight Forum on Drugs, Ireland 82–3

P
Poland 89, 90–2, 202–3
policies, public 1–8
  classification 11–17, 26
  cluster analysis 22–4
  common features in EU member states 42–3
  EU *see* European Union (EU) policy
  historical context 3–6

policy factors 19, 20
  codified variables 143–4
  variables and their definitions 151–7
Pompidou Group of the Council of Europe 42
Portugal 61–4, 129, 204–5
poverty rate, at-risk 150
prevention
  model 1 countries 52, 54, 57–8, 61, 63–4, 65
  model 2 countries 72–4, 77, 79–80, 84
  model 3 countries 91, 92, 94, 99
  model 4 countries 113, 115–16
prime ministers 103, 106
Program Domowych programme 91
public-health approach 4–5, 121, 140

Q
quality of life assessment 10
'Quit the Shit' programme 52

R
Ramon, A. xv
RAND Europe 38
recreational drug use 5
regulation of legal substances model *see*
  model 2
relational management strategy *see* well-being
  and relational management strategy
research methodology *see* methodology,
  research
Romania 103, 115–16, 206–7

S
safety and disease approach 19, 21
  model 1 countries 55
  model 3 countries 93, 95, 96, 97
  model 4 countries 106, 110–11, 114, 115
Schengen Agreement (1985) 30, 35–6, 44
school-based programmes
  model 1 countries 52, 54, 58, 64
  model 3 countries 94, 99
Searching Family Treasure programme 64
Segura, L. xv
Silk Route, drug trafficking 39, 112
similarity measure, Gower's 22
Slovakia 105–7, 208–9
Slovenia 89, 98–100, 210–11
smoking *see* tobacco consumption
smuggling, tobacco 40, 82
Spain 65–7, 212–13
SpiritsEUROPE 37
stakeholder participation
  different member states 122–3
  EU policy-making 36–8, 123
state factors 19, 20
  codified variables 143
  variables and definitions 145–50
status index 10, 146
Stewart-Clark Committee report (1986) 30

Stiglitz Commission 10
stigmatization, heroin users 5
strategy domain 19–20, 21, 123
  cluster analysis 22, 23
  codified variables 144
  model 2 countries 72
  operationalization of variables 139–40
  variables and their definitions 157–60
structure domain 20–2, 123
  cluster analysis 22, 23
  codified variables 144
  operationalization of variables 140–2
  variables and their definitions 160–1
substance-based reactive intervention
  approach 20–2
Suchtmittelgesetz (SMG), Austria 92–3
supply reduction 17, 140
  EU policies 34–5, 43
  model 2 countries 72, 79–80, 81–2, 83–4
  model 4 countries 105, 115
sustainable governance indicators 10, 12–13
Sweden 69, 74–7, 214–15
  influence on EU policies 32, 34
syringe exchange *see* needle and syringe
  exchange
Systembolaget, Sweden 76

T
Tampere Summit 34
television advertising 31
temperance movements 4, 78
tobacco
  geopolitics 40
  smuggling 40, 82
tobacco consumption (smoking)
  deaths related to 2, 40
  European countries 71
  model 1 countries 53, 56, 57, 66
  model 2 countries 70, 78
  model 4 countries 105, 110
  variables 152
tobacco-control scale 16, 140, 159
  European countries 73
  model 1 countries 57, 58, 65
  model 2 countries 76, 78, 82
  model 3 countries 90, 93, 95, 100
  model 4 countries 105, 111, 113, 116
tobacco-free by 2040 initiative, Finland
  78, 79
tobacco industry 37, 40
tobacco policy and control
  classification 14, 16–17
  EU 31, 32–4, 35, 40
  France 80, 81
  Luxembourg 59
  model 4 countries 107
  role of civil society groups 37–8
  role of international organizations 41–2

traditional approach *see* model 4
trajectory, governance of addictions 142
transitioning model *see* model 3
transversality 141
treatment
  model 1 countries 56, 59, 60, 61
  model 2 countries 72–4
  model 3 countries 94, 96
  model 4 countries 109, 110
trendsetters in illicit substances model *see*
  model 1
Trevi Group 30
Turkey 39

U
unemployment rate 149–50
United Kingdom (UK) 83–5, 216–17
  minimum unit pricing for alcohol 84
  substance consumption 69, 71
United Nations (UN) 41
United Nations (UN) Convention Against
  Illicit Traffic in Narcotic Drugs and
  Psychotropic Substances (1988) 4, 30–1,
  156
United Nations (UN) Convention on
  Psychotropic Substances (1971) 30, 156
United Nations General Assembly, 1988
  Special Session (UNGASS) 32

United Nations Office on Drugs and Crime
  (UNODC) 41
United Nations (UN) Single Convention on
  Narcotic Drugs (1961) and Protocol
  (1972) 4, 30, 155–6

W
welfare state regimes, Esping-Andersen 9–10,
  12–13, 126–7
well-being
  measuring 10
  as national objective 95, 114–15
  in national strategy 121, 140
well-being and relational management
    strategy 20, 21
  model 1 countries 47–8, 55, 67–8
  model 2 countries 71, 72
  model 3 countries 90, 95
wicked social problems 6–7
World Health Organization (WHO) 41–2
  definition of addiction 2
  Framework Convention on Tobacco Control
    (FCTC) 35, 41–2, 155
World Values Survey, Inglehart 11, 12–13,
  147–8

Y
Ysa, T. xv